2019–20 Peripheral Brain for the
PHARMACIST

Jeanine P. Abrons, PharmD, MS

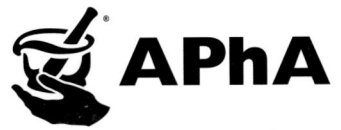

Washington, DC

Acquiring Editor: Janan Sarwar
Managing Editors: John Fedor and Janan Sarwar
Project Manager: Ashley Young, Publications Professionals LLC
Copyeditors: Connie Moy and Ashley Young, Publications Professionals LLC
Composition: Circle Graphics, Inc.
Cover Design: Michelle Powell, APhA Integrated Design and
Production Center

Published by the American Pharmacists Association,
2215 Constitution Avenue, NW, Washington, DC 20037-2985
www.pharmacist.com • www.pharmacylibrary.com

To comment on this product by email, send your message to the publisher
at *aphabooks@aphanet.org.*

Library of Congress Cataloging-in-Publication Data

Names: Abrons, Jeanine P., editor. | American Pharmacists Association,
  issuing body.
Title: Peripheral brain for the pharmacist / edited by Jeanine P. Abrons.
Description: 2019-2020 edition. | Washington, DC : American Pharmacists
  Association, [2019]
Identifiers: LCCN 2019006084 | ISBN 9781582123158
Subjects: | MESH: Pharmaceutical Preparations | Drug Therapy | Handbook
Classification: LCC RM301 | NLM QV 39 | DDC 615.1--dc23 LC record
available at https://lccn.loc.gov/2019006084

How to Order This Product

Online: www.pharmacist.com/shop
By phone: 800-878-0729 (770-250-0085 from outside the
U.S. and Canada)
VISA®, MasterCard®, and American Express® cards accepted.

Contents

CARDIOLOGY

Hypertension Management 1
Atherosclerotic Cardiovascular Disease (ASCVD) Risk **(NEW)** 5
Associated Lipid Goals Based Upon Level of Risk—AACE Guidelines 8
Selection of Statin Intensity-Based ASCVD Risk in Patients
 with Diabetes 8
Cholesterol Management: Use of Drug Classes
 Other than Statins **(NEW)** 9
Direct Oral Anticoagulants **(NEW)** 11
Injectable Anticoagulants 13
Perioperative Management of Direct Oral Anticoagulants 16
Common Warfarin Drug Interactions 17
Warfarin Dosing According to the 9th Edition of CHEST Guidelines 18
Alterations to Warfarin Dose Maintenance Therapy 20

ENDOCRINOLOGY

Diabetes Treatment Guidelines **(NEW)** 22
Goals of Care for Patients with Diabetes 23
Associated Goals for Adults with Diabetes **(NEW)** 24
Insulin and Insulin Analogues 25
Management of Type 2 Diabetes **(NEW)** 26
Injectable Type 2 Diabetes Medications 28

RESPIRATORY

Initiating Therapy in Children with Intermittent Asthma Severity 29
Initiating Therapy in Children with Persistent Asthma Severity 30
Adjusting Asthma Therapy in Children Ages 0 to 4 31
Adjusting Asthma Therapy in Children Ages 5 to 11 32
Stepwise Approach for Managing Asthma Long Term
 in Children Ages 0 to 4 33
Stepwise Approach for Managing Asthma Long Term
 in Children Ages 5 to 11 33
Initiating Therapy in Youths ≥ 12 Years of Age and Adults
 with Intermittent Asthma Severity 34
Initiating Therapy in Youths ≥ 12 Years of Age and Adults
 with Persistent Asthma Severity 35
Assessing Therapy in Youths ≥ 12 Years of Age and Adults
 Based on Asthma Control 36
Stepwise Approach for Managing Asthma Long Term
 in Youths ≥ 12 Years of Age and Adults 36
Assessment of Airflow Limitation/Symptoms in Chronic
 Obstructive Pulmonary Disease (COPD) 37
Assessment to Determine ABCD Groups in Chronic Obstructive
 Pulmonary Disease (COPD) 38

Contents

INFECTIOUS DISEASES

Community-Acquired Pneumonia (CAP) Management 39
Treatment of Community-Acquired Pneumonia (CAP). 40
Hospital-Acquired Pneumonia (HAP) Management 41
Aminoglycosides: Traditional Considerations and Dosing in Adults 43
Aminoglycosides: Single Daily Dosing 44
Vancomycin: Considerations and Dosing in Adults 45
Vancomycin: General Information and Dosing (PO/IV) for
  C. difficile Colitis **(NEW)** 46
Gram Stain Interpretation – GRAM + RESULT **(NEW)** 47
Gram Stain Interpretation – GRAM – RESULT **(NEW)** 48
Consideration of When to Draw Cultures vs. Start Antibiotics
  in the Emergency Department (ED) **(NEW)** 49
Consider Whether to Draw a Culture (General) **(NEW)**. 50

SPECIAL POPULATIONS
Pediatric
Usual Pediatric Dosages of Common Over-the-Counter (OTC)
  Medications 51
Pediatric Commercially Available Dosage Forms and Doses/
  Concentrations of Analgesics 52
Pediatric Commercially Available Dosage Forms and Doses/
  Concentrations of Antihistamines. 53
Pediatric Commercially Available Dosage Forms and Doses
  for Antiflatulents. 54
Pediatric Measurements. 54
Geriatric
Inappropriate Medications in Older Adults 55
Women's Health
Pregnancy and Lactation Resources 57
Pregnancy Risk Classifications 58
Safe and Unsafe Use of OTC Medications during Pregnancy 59

IMMUNIZATIONS (UPDATED ANNUALLY)
Immunization Schedule for Children and Adults Ages 18 Years
  or Younger 60
Immunizations by Age for First Year of Life. 62
2018 Recommended Immunizations for Children from Birth
  Through 6 Years Old **(NEW)**. 63
Travel Immunization and Travel Health Card 64

Contents

CALCULATIONS/CONVERSIONS/GENERAL MONITORING

Calculations

Ideal Body Weight (IBW)..68

Body Mass Index (BMI)..68

Creatinine Clearance Calculations....................................69

Conversions

Conversions 70

Weights and Measures..71

Apothecary Equivalents...72

Opioid Conversions..73

Systemic Corticosteroid Conversions 74

Monitoring

Target Serum Concentrations for Selected Drugs 75

Normal Laboratory Values 76

Fluid Composition and Calculations 78

Electrolytes and Minerals...79

SPECIFIC DISEASE STATE MANAGEMENT

Psychiatry Guidelines...80

Psychiatric Medications...81

Nutrition..82

Chronic Kidney Disease...87

Acute Pain Management 88

Veterinary Medicine Information 89

MISCELLANEOUS

Quality, Free Online Resources 90

National Clinical Guidelines 91

Clinically Significant Drug Interactions 93

Medications with Adverse Withdrawal Effects
  from Abrupt Discontinuation 94

FASTHUG-MAIDENS: Approach to Identifying Drug-Related
  Problems (DRPs) & Aspects of Critical Care for
  Intensive Care Units (ICU) Pharmacists **(NEW)** 97

Pharmacy Mnemonics..99

COUNSELING AND STANDARDS OF CARE

Motivational Interviewing Techniques............................100

Pharmacists' Patient Care Process..............................101

Call for Ideas

Submit ideas for new cards in future editions of the *Peripheral Brain*.
Send your ideas to aphabooks@aphanet.org. Thanks!

Please let us know the most useful content or additional areas that
you'd like to see in the future to further increase the value of this product.

Contributors

AUTHORS

JEANINE P. ABRONS, PharmD, MS
Clinical Assistant Professor/Director of
  Student Pharmacists International Activities
University of Iowa College of Pharmacy
Iowa City, Iowa

ELISHA ANDREAS, PharmD
Pharmacist
Hartig Drug
Iowa City, Iowa

JENNA BLUNT
Postgraduate Year 2 Resident
John Hopkins Medicine
Baltimore, Maryland

MARK BOTTI, PharmD, BCPPS, AE-C
Pharmacist
Albany Medical Center
Albany, New York

SARA E. DUGAN, PharmD, BCPP, BCPS
Associate Professor of Pharmacy Practice
Northeast Ohio Medical University
  College of Pharmacy
Rootstown, Ohio

BRITTANY HAYES, BS, RRT, RCP, PharmD
Post Graduate Year 2 Resident
Veterans Affairs Medical Center-
Tennessee Valley Healthcare System
Nashville, Tennessee

STEVEN HONG
PharmD Candidate 2019
University of Iowa, College of Pharmacy
Iowa City, Iowa

BEN LOMAESTRO, PharmD
Senior Clinical Pharmacy Specialist–
  Infectious Disease
Albany Medical Center
Albany, New York

ANH LUONG, PharmD
Des Moines, Iowa

VERN DUBA, MA
Clinical Assistant Professor
University of Iowa College of Pharmacy
Iowa City, Iowa

NICOLE BUCCI, PharmD
Post Graduate Year 1 Resident
Albany Medical Center
Albany, New York

SHAWN PHILLIPS
Post Graduate Year 1 Resident
Albany Medical Center
Albany, New York

ERICA MACEIRA, PharmD, BCPS, CACP
Clinical Pharmacy Specialist
Transplant and Anticoagulation
Albany Medical Center
Albany, New York

JASMINE MANGRUM
PharmD Candidate 2019
University of Iowa College of Pharmacy
Iowa City, Iowa

REBECCA PETRIK, PharmD
Clinical Pharmacist
UC Health University of Colorado Hospital
Aurora, CO

MOLLY HENRY, PharmD
Solid Organ Transplant Clinical Pharmacist
The University of Kansas Health System
Kansas City, MO

JESSICA RAMICH, PharmD
Clinical Pharmacy Specialist
Guthrie Corning Hospital
Big Flats, New York

ADRIENNE ROUILLER, PharmD
Clinical Pharmacist
Health Alliance Hospital
Leominster, Massachusetts

JOANNA RUSCH, PharmD
Post Graduate Year 1 Resident
Mann-Grandstaff Veterans Affairs Medical Center
Spokane, WA

BREANNA SUNDERMAN, PharmD
Pharmacist, HyVee Pharmacy
Clarinda, Iowa

BRYAN PINCKNEY WHITE, PharmD, BCPS
Infectious Diseases Clinical Pharmacist
Oklahoma University Medical Center
Oklahoma City, OKlahoma

ANGELA WOJTCZAK, PharmD
Community-based Post Graduate Year 1 Resident
North Shore University Health System
Northbrook, IL

ANASTASIA LUNDT, PharmD
Clinical Pharmacist, University of Iowa Hospitals
  and Clinics
Iowa City, Iowa

Acknowledgments

The editor and publisher gratefully acknowledge Jennifer Cerulli, PharmD, BCPS, and Renée Ahrens Thomas, PharmD, MBA, for their help in selecting the contents of previous editions; and Jennifer L. Adams, PharmD, EdD, and Keith D. Marciniak, BSPharm, who developed the concept of reference cards in an APhA resource that preceded *Peripheral Brain for the Pharmacist*. The editor and publisher gratefully recognize Alecia Heh for her involvement in previous versions of Diabetes related pages, and Eric P. Boateng for his work on the Medications with Adverse Withdrawal Effects from Abrupt Discontinuation pages.

Reviewers

KELLI COVINGTON, PharmD, BCPPS, BCPS
Assistant Professor of Clinical Sciences/
  Pediatric Pharmacy Clinical Specialist
Roosevelt University College of Pharmacy
Chicago, IL

LESLIE HAMILTON, PharmD, FCCP, FCCM, BCPS, BCCCP
Associate Professor of Clinical Pharmacy and
  Translational Science
University of Tennessee Health Science Center
  College of Pharmacy
Knoxville, TN

TROY LYNN LEWIS, PharmD
Assistant Professor of Pharmacy Practice
Wilkes University Nesbitt School of Pharmacy
Wilkes-Barre, PA

SHAINA MUSCO, PharmD
Assistant Professor of Clinical Sciences
High Point University Fred Wilson School of Pharmacy
High Point, NC

MICHELE RICCARDI, PharmD, BCPS
Assistant Professor of Pharmacy Practice and
  Administration
University of St. Joseph School of Pharmacy
  and Physician Assistant Studies
West Hartford, CT

BENJAMIN SCOTT, PharmD
Clinical Pharmacist Educator
University of Kentucky Healthcare
Lexington, KY

SNEHA BAXI SRIVASTAVA, PharmD, BCACP, CDE
Associate Professor
Rosalind Franklin University College of Pharmacy
North Chicago, IL

MALLORY TURNER, PharmD, BCPS
Assistant Professor, Pharmacy Practice
Harding University College of Pharmacy
Searcy, AR

CUCNHAT WALKER, PharmD, BCPS, MPH
Assistant Clinical Professor
Larkin University
Miami, FL

JORDAN WULZ, PharmD, MPH, BC-ADM
Assistant Professor of Pharmacy Practice
Concordia University Wisconsin
Mequon, WI

Hypertension Management

High Blood Pressure Guideline Summary: The 2017 Guideline for the Prevention, Detection, Evaluation, & Management of High Blood Pressure in Adults represents an update of the Joint National Committee (JNC) guidelines from 2003. The guidelines include information from studies on related risk of CVD & monitoring, & include thresholds to start drug treatment & goals.

Classifying High Blood Pressure (BP) in Adults

CATEGORY	SYSTOLIC Blood Pressure (SBP) in mmHg		DIASTOLIC Blood Pressure (DBP) in mmHg
Normal	< 120	AND	< 80
Elevated	120–129	AND	< 80
Hypertension (HTN) • Stage 1 • Stage 2	130–139 ≥ 140	OR OR	80–89 ≥ 90

Patient with high SBP & DBP in 2 categories: select the higher category.
Caution: BP is based on an average of ≥ 2 readings taken on ≥ 2 occasions.
BP measurements in clinical trial may not represent typical level of care & patient motivation.

Use of CVD Risk Estimation* and Blood Pressure Threshold to Guide Drug Treatment
Use of BP-lowering medications are recommended for:
• ***Primary prevention*** of CVD for patients with no history of CVD **AND** 10-year ASCVD risk < 10% & SBP ≥ 140 mmHg or DBP ≥ 90 mmHg   • ***Primary prevention*** of CVD for patients with 10-year ASCVD risk ≥ 10% & average SBP ≥ 130 mmHg or average DBP ≥ 80 mmHg   • ***Secondary prevention*** of recurrent CVD events for patients with clinical CVD & average SBP ≥ 130 mmHg or average DBP ≥ 80 mmHg
Initial Monotherapy Versus Initial Combination Drug Therapy
• ***Stage 1 hypertension (HTN) & BP goal < 130/80 mmHg***:   Start 1 antihypertensive drug. Titrate dose & sequentially add other agents to achieve BP target.   • ***Stage 2 hypertension & average BP > 20/10 mmHg above target***:   Start 2 first-line agents of different classes, either as separate agents or in fixed-dose combination.
Initial Medication Options
• ***First-line agents***: ACE or ARB, thiazide diuretics, & CCB

*Notes: *ACC/AHA Risk Estimator Plus: http://tools.acc.org/ASCVD-Risk-Estimator-Plus/ (Accessed 2018); ASCVD was defined as a first congenital heart disease death, nonfatal myocardial infarction or nonfatal stroke. CVD = cardiovascular disease; ASCVD = atherosclerotic cardiovascular disease; ACE = angiotensin conversion enzyme inhibitor; ARB = angiotensin receptor blocker; CCB = calcium channel blocker.*

Hypertension Management *(continued)*

Considerations in Care – Management of High Blood Pressure

CONSIDERATION	DESCRIPTION	
Blood Pressure Management	• Accurate management is critical. • Consider out-of-office & self-monitoring to confirm & titrate medications. • Measurement values may vary depending on time & location taken.	
Screen/Manage Other CVD Risk Factors	• Smoking; diabetes; dyslipidemia; weight; low fitness; poor diet; stress; sleep apnea • Testing	
	BASIC testing	Complete blood count; fasting blood glucose; lipid profile; serum creatinine with estimated glomerular filtration rate (eGFR); serum electrolytes (K^+; Na^{2+}; Ca^{2+}); thyroid-stimulating hormone (TSH); urinalysis; electrocardiogram
	OPTIONAL testing	Echocardiogram; uric acid; urine albumin to creatinine ratio
Screen for Secondary Causes of HTN	• Screen for common secondary causes with new-onset or uncontrolled hypertension. • If more specific clinical symptoms are present, consider uncommon secondary causes.	
	What to Screen For	
	COMMON Causes to prompt need to	
	Screen for secondary causes of hypertension Primary aldosteronism (elevated aldosterone/renin ratio) CKD (chronic kidney disease) (eGFR < 60 mL/min/1.73 m²) Renal artery stenosis (young female, known atherosclerotic disease, worsening kidney function) Obstructive sleep apnea (snoring, witnessed apnea, excessive daytime sleepiness)	• Abrupt onset • Age < 30 • Drug resistant/induced: uncontrolled BP after treatment with ≥ 3 antihypertensives • Excessive target organ damage (e.g., cerebral vascular disease; retinopathy; left ventricular hypertrophy, heart failure [HF] with preserved ejection fraction [EF] or with reserved EF; coronary artery disease [CAD]; chronic kidney disease; peripheral artery disease; albuminuria) • OR onset of diastolic HTN in older adults • OR unprovoked or excessive hypokalemia
	UNCOMMON Causes **(< 1%)**	• Acromegaly • Aortic coarctation • Congenital adrenal hyperplasia • Mineralocorticoid excess syndrome (not primary aldosteronism) • Cushing syndrome • Hypo-hyperthyroidism or primary hyperparathyroidism • Phenochromocytoma/paraganglioma
Follow-up	**ADULT PATIENT GROUP**	**FREQUENCY OF FOLLOW-UP**
	Low risk with elevated BP or stage 1 HTN with ASCVD risk < 10%	Repeat BP after 3 to 6 months of nonpharmacological therapy
	Stage 1 HTN & high ASCVD risk (≥ 10% 10-year ASCVD risk)	Repeat BP after 1 month of nonpharmacologic & antihypertensive drug therapy
	Stage 2 HTN	Evaluate by primary care provider (PCP) within 1 month of diagnosis; treat with combo of non-pharmacologic & 2 antihypertensive drugs from different classes; repeat evaluation in 1 month
	Very high average BP (systolic ≥ 160 mmHg or diastolic ≥ 100 mmHg)	Evaluate promptly; monitor carefully & adjust dose upward as needed
	Normal BP	Repeat BP evaluation annually

Causes of Drug-Induced Elevations in Blood Pressure

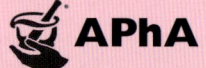

Hypertension Management *(continued)*

Type of Medication	Medication	Recommendation
NON-PRESCRIPTION	**Alcohol**	• Limit to ≤ 1 drink (women); ≤ 2 drinks (men).
	Caffeine	• Limit to < 300 mg/day. • Avoid in uncontrolled HTN. • May only have acute effect on BP.
	Decongestants (phenylephrine; pseudoephedrine)	• Use for short duration. • Avoid in severe or uncontrolled HTN. • Consider alternative.
	Herbals (ephedra [ma-huang]; St. John's Wort with MAOIs* and yohimbine)	• Avoid use.
	Illicit Drug Use (cocaine; methamphetamine)	• Avoid use.
	Nonsteroidal Anti-Inflammatory Agents (NSAIDs)	• Avoid use. • Consider alternative analgesic.
PRESCRIPTION	**Antidepressants** (MAOIs*; SNRIs;** TCAs***)	• Consider alternatives (selective seratonin reuptake inhibitors [SSRIs]). • Avoid tyramine containing foods if on MAOIs*.
	Amphetamines (amphetamine; methylphenidate; dexmethylphenidate; dextroamphetamine)	• Discontinue or decrease dose. • Consider alternatives (behavioral therapy).
	Atypical Antipsychotics (clozapine; olanzapine)	• Discontinue or limit use. • Consider alternatives (behavioral therapy; lifestyle modifications; other agents [with less weight gain, diabetes or dyslipidemia risk]; e.g., aripiprazole; ziprasidone).
	Oral Contraceptives	• Use low-dose estrogens (20 to 30 mcg ethinyl estradiol) or progestin only. • Consider alternatives (e.g., barrier method; abstinence; intrauterine devices [IUD]). • Avoid in uncontrolled HTN.
	Immunosuppressants (cyclosporine)	• Consider changing to tacrolimus, which may be associated with fewer BP effects.
	Systemic corticosteroids	• Avoid or limit use if possible. • Consider other routes (inhaled, topical) when feasible.

*Notes: *MAOI = monoamine oxidase inhibitors; **SNRIs = seratonin norepinephrine reuptake inhibitors; ***TCA = tricyclic antidepressants.*

Hypertension Management *(continued)*

Management of High Blood Pressure in Specific Patient Populations

Population	Additional Description of Population	Target Blood Pressure (BP) or Recommended Treatment
Adults	Confirmed HTN* & known cardiovascular disease (CVD) or 10-year ASCVD** risk > 10%	< 130/80 mmHg
	Confirmed HTN without added markers of ↑ CVD risk	< 130/80 mmHg
Older Persons (> 65 years old)	Noninstitutionalized ambulatory community-dwelling adults with average systolic BP (SBP) ≥ 130 mmHg	< 130 mmHg
	HTN + high burden of comorbidity + limited life expectancy	Clinical judgment, patient preference, & team-based care; consider risk/benefit for decisions on intensity of BP ↓ & antihypertensive drugs
Hypertensive Adults + Heart Failure (HF) Risk	To prevent HF in hypertensive adults	< 130/80 mmHg
Hypertension + HFrEF	GDMT*** titrated to BP	< 130/80 mmHg Nondihydropyridine calcium channel blockers (CCBs) not recommended
Hypertension + HFpEF	Volume overload	Control HTN with diuretics
	HFpEF & persistent HTN after volume overload is managed	Angiotensin-converting enzyme inhibitors (ACE [-]) or angiotensin receptor blockers (ARBs) & beta blockers; titrate to SBP < 130 mmHg
Hypertension + CKD	HTN + CKD	< 130/80 mmHg
	HTN + CKD Stage ≥ 3 OR Stage 1 or 2 + albuminuria (≥ 300 mg/d, OR ≥ 300 mg/g albumin-to-creatinine ratio OR equivalent in 1st morning void)	ACE (-) to slow CKD progression or an ARB if ACE (-) intolerant
Hypertension + DM	BP ≥ 130/80 mmHg	Start antihypertensive drug to goal of < 130/80 mmHg; ACE (-), ARBs, diuretics, & CCBs = effective
	With albuminuria	ACE (-) or ARBs
Race and Ethnicity	Black adults with HTN but no HF or CKD, + DM	Thiazide-type diuretic or CCB for initial treatment
	Hypertensive adults, especially black adults	≥ 2 antihypertensives to achieve target of < 130/80 mmHg

*Notes: *hypertension; **atherosclerotic cardiovascular disease; ***guideline-directed medication therapy; HFrEF = heart failure with reduced ejection fraction; HFpEF = heart failure with preserved ejection fraction; CKD = chronic kidney disease; DM = diabetes mellitus.*

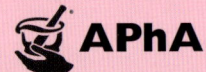

Atherosclerotic Cardiovascular Disease (ASCVD) Risk

ASCVD Risk Estimation Calculator:
http://tools.acc.org/ascvd-risk-estimator-plus/#!/calculate/estimate/ (Accessed 2018)

Other Potential Scoring Systems for Cardiovascular Risk

Scoring System	Notes on Scoring System	Calculator or Additional Information Available
Framingham	• Intended for use in nondiabetic patients 30–79 years old with no history of coronary heart disease or intermittent claudication • Most widely applicable to patients without previous cardiac disease	• https://www.framinghamheartstudy.org/fhs-risk-functions/cardiovascular-disease-10-year-risk/
Multi-Ethnic Study of Atherosclerosis (MESA)	• Most appropriate for patients 45–85 years old and in the following racial/ethnic groups: Caucasian, Chinese American, African American, or Hispanic	• https://mesa-nhlbi.org/MESACHDRisk/MesaRiskScore/RiskScore.aspx
Reynolds Risk Score for Cardiovascular Risk	• For women > 45 years old	• http://www.reynoldsriskscore.org
UK Prospective Diabetes Study (UKPDS) Risk	• Scoring system for type 2 diabetes	• https://www.dtu.ox.ac.uk/riskengine/

Note: All websites accessed 2018.

Risk Factors for Atherosclerotic Cardiovascular Disease

Major Risk Factors	Other (Additional or Nontraditional)
• ↑ Age • ↑ Serum cholesterol • ↑ Non-HDL • ↑ LDL-C • Low HDL-C • Diabetes mellitus • Hypertension • Chronic kidney disease • Cigarette smoking • Family history of ASCVD	• Obesity/abdominal obesity • Family history of hyperlipidemia • ↑ small, dense LDL-C • ↑ Apo-lipoprotein B • ↑ LDL particle concentration • Fasting/postprandial hypertriglyeridemia • PCOS • Dyslipidemic triad* • ↑ Lipoprotein (a) • ↑ Clotting factors • ↑ Inflammatory markers (hsCRP; Lp-PLA$_2$)

Notes: HDL = high-density lipoprotein; LDL = low-density lipoprotein; C = cholesterol; ASCVD = atherosclerotic cardiovascular disease; PCOS = polycystic ovarian syndrome; hsCRP = high sensitive C-reactive protein; Lp-PLA$_2$ = lipoprotein-associated phospholipase. * = hypertriglyceridemia (triglycerides >150 mg/dL); low high-density lipoprotein cholesterol (HDL-C; ≤ 35 mg/dL); and small, dense low-density lipoprotein particles.

Reference: Modified from Table 6 – Clinical Practice Guidelines for Managing Dyslidemia & Prevention of CVD, Endocr Pract. 2017;23(Suppl 2) 17 Copyright © 2017 AACE.

Atherosclerotic Cardiovascular Disease (ASCVD) Risk *(continued)*

Steps to Determine Management Strategy to Reduce Lipids and Risk of Atherosclerotic Cardiovascular Disease

Step #	Overall Step	Description of Step			
1	Determine ASCVD risk.	• Use a scoring system for cardiovascular risk, determine if the patient does or does not have clinical ASCVD, and/or measure a coronary artery calcium score.			
2	Encourage a healthy lifestyle.	• Individualize lifestyle modifications to each patient. • May include smoking cessation, diet modification, physical activity, and weight reduction to target an optimal weight.			
3	Consider medications.	• Discuss selection of lipid-lowering medications including benefit/risk/cost analysis. • As ASCVD risk ↑ benefits of evidence-based lipid-lowering medications also ↑.			
4	If treatment favors lipid-lowering medications, use evidence-based medicine. (Assess ASCVD risk by age group & emphasize adherence to healthy lifestyle.)	**Primary Prevention**		**Secondary Prevention** (refer to page 8 for definitions)		
		Patient Factor	Recommendation	ASCVD not at very high risk	Very high risk ASCVD	

		LDL-C ≥ 190 mg/dL	• No risk assessment; use high-intensity statin	• For age ≤75 years old, use high-intensity statin with a goal LDL-C ↓ of ≤ 50%.
				  o If high-intensity statin not tolerated, use moderate-intensity statin
				• If on max statin therapy & LDL-C ≥ 70 mg/dL + may add ezetimibe
				• For age > 75 years old: reasonable to initiate moderate- or high-intensity statin OR continuation of high-intensity statin is reasonable
					• Use high-intensity or maximal statin:
					  o If on max statin & LDL-C ≥ 70 mg/dL + may add ezetimibe
					  o If PCS9-I is considered, add ezetimibe to max statin before + PCSK9-I
					  o If on max LDL-C↓ therapy & LDL-C ≥70 mg/dL or non-HDL-C ≥100 mg/dL may + PCSK9-I	

		Diabetes & age 40–75 years old:	• Moderate-intensity statin • Risk assessment to consider high-intensity statin			
		Age 0–19 years old	• Lifestyle modifications to ↓ ASCVD risk • With diagnosis of familial hypercholesterolemia: statin			
		Age 20–39 years old	• Lifetime risk estimation • Consider statin if family history (FH) or premature ASCVD & LDL-C > 160 mg/dL			
		Age 40–75 years old without diabetes and LDL 70 to 18mg/dL	• For all risk levels, discuss risk ↓ • Risk 5 – < 7.5%: may + moderate intensity statin • Risk ≥ 7.5 – < 20%: may + moderate intensity statin to ↓ LDL-C by 30–49% ≥ 20%: + statin to ↓ LDL-C by ≥50% < 5%: emphasize lifestyle to reduce risk factors			
		Age > 75 years old	• Clinical assessment & risk discussion			
5	Regularly reasses.	• Frequently evaluate patient goals for ASCVD risk ↓, medication tolerability/affordability, and treatment plans.			

Note: LDL-C = low-density lipoprotein cholesterol; non-HDL = non-high-density lipoprotein; PCKS9-1 = proprotein convertase subtilisin/kexin type 9 serine protease inhibitor.

References: Table modified from: Krumholz HM. Treatment of Cholesterol in 2017. JAMA. 2017;318(5):417–418. Doi:10.1001/jama.2017.6753. Available at: https://jamanetwork.com/journals/jama/article-abstract/2645740 (Accessed November 2018); Figure 1: Secondary Prevention in Patients with Clinical ASCVD & Figure 2: Primary Prevention in Grundy SM, Stone NJ, Bailey AL, Beam C, Birtcher KK et al. 2018–AHA/ACC/AACVPR/AAPA/ACPM/ADA/AGS/AphA/ASPC/NLA/PCNA Guideline on the Management of Blood Cholesterol. A Report to the American College of Cardiology/American Heart Association Task Force on Clinical Practice Guidelines. Circulation. 2018. Available at: https://www.ahajournals.org/doi/abs/10.1161/CIR.0000000000000625 (Accessed November 2018).

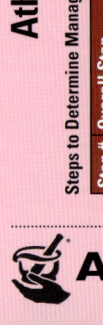

Atherosclerotic Cardiovascular Disease (ASCVD) Risk *(continued)*

Process of Evaluating a Patient Prior to Initiation of a Statin:

Initial evaluation prior to statin initiation:

- Fasting lipid panel
- Alanine aminotransferase
- Creatinine Kinase (CK) [If indicated]
- Hemoglobin A1c [If diabetes status unknown]
- Consider evaluation for other secondary causes or conditions that may influence statin safety

Treat Laboratory Abnormalities

- Triglycerides ≥ 500 mg/dL
- LDL-C ≥ 190 mg/dL
- Unexplained ALT ≥ 3 x the Upper Limit of Normal (ULN)

Other Biomarker Monitoring with Cholesterol Management:

Biomarker	Notes
Coronary artery calcium (CAC)	• Consider monitoring if risk decision is unknown • Interpretation: **CAC Value** / **Interpretation** **0** — Lower risk; consider no statin, unless diabetic, family history (FH) of premature coronary heart disease (CHD), or cigarette smoker **1–99** — Favors statin use (especially after age 55) **100+ &/or ≥ 75th percentile** — Initiate statin therapy
High-sensitivity C-reactive protein (Hs-CRP)	• Inflammatory marker • Elevation = ≥ 2 mg/dL • Measure with persistently elevated triglycerides (TG) ≥ 175 mg/dL
Ankle-brachial index (ABI)	• Ratio of blood pressure (BP) at the ankle to BP in the brachium • Compared to arm, lower BP in the leg suggests blocked artery secondary to peripheral artery disease (PAD) • Measure with persistently elevated TG ≥ 175 mg/dL
Lipoprotein a	• Relative indicator for measurement = FH of premature atherosclerotic coronary artery disease (ASCVD) • Measure with persistently elevated triglycerides (TG) ≥ 175 mg/dL

Reference: Based on recommendations from Grundy SM, Stone NJ, Bailey AL, Beam C, Birtcher KK et al. 2018–AHA/ACC/AACVPR/AAPA/ACPM/ADA/AGS/AphA/ASPC/NLA/PCNA Guideline on the Management of Blood Cholesterol. A Report to the American College of Cardiology/American Heart Association Task Force on Clinical Practice Guidelines. Circulation, 2018. Available at: https://www.ahajournals.org/doi/abs/10.1161/CIR.0000000000000625 (Accessed November 2018).

Associated Lipid Goals Based Upon Level of Risk— AACE Guidelines

Level of Risk	Risk Factors/10-year Risk	Treatment Goals (In mg/dL)
Extreme	• Progressive ASCVD including UA after achieving LDL-C < 70 mg/dL • Established clinical cardiovascular disease in patients with DM, CKD (Stage 3 or 4), or HeFH • History of premature ASCVD (males: < 55; females: < 65)	LDL-C < 55; HDL-C < 80; ApoB < 70
Very High	• Established or recent hospitalization (for ACS; coronary, carotid, or PVD) or 10-year risk > 20% • Diabetes or CKD (Stage 3 or 4) with 1+ risk factor • HeFH	LDL-C < 70; HDL-C: < 100; ApoB < 80
High	• ≥ 2 risk factor & 10-year risk = 10–20% • Diabetes or CKD (Stage 3 or 4) with no other risk factors	LDL-C < 100; HDL-C < 130; ApoB < 90
Moderate	• ≤ 2 risk factors & 10-year risk < 10%	LDL-C < 100; HDL-C < 130; ApoB
Low	• 0 risk factors	LDL-C < 130; HDL-C < 160; ApoB = NR

Notes: UA = unstable angina; LDL-C = low-density lipoprotein cholesterol; HDL-C = high-density lipoprotein cholesterol; DM = diabetes mellitus; CKD = chronic kidney disease; HeFH = familial hypercholesterolemia; ACS = acute coronary syndrome; PVD = peripheral vascular disease; AACE = American Association of Clinical Endocrinologists; NR = not recommended.

Reference: Modified from Table 6 – Clinical Practice Guidelines for Managing Dyslipidemia & Prevention of CVD, Endocr Pract. 2017;23(Suppl 2) 17 Copyright © 2017 AACE.

Prepared by Erica Maceira and Jeanine Abrons

Selection of Statin Intensity-Based ASCVD Risk in Patients with Diabetes

Age	No Known Risk Factors	ASCVD Risk Factor(s)*	ASCVD
< 40	No statin therapy	Moderate- or high-intensity statin	High-intensity statin
40-75	Moderate-intensity statin	High-intensity statin	High-intensity statin
> 75[a]	Moderate-intensity statin	Moderate- or high-intensity statin	High-intensity statin

a: If patient has change to acute coronary syndrome (ACS) and LDL cholesterol > 50 mg/dL and cannot tolerate high-dose statins, consider moderate-intensity statin dosing plus the addition of ezetimibe.

*ASCVD risk factors include low-density lipoprotein (LDL) ≥ 100 mg/dL, high blood pressure, smoking, overweight or obesity, and family history of premature ASCVD.

Notes:
- *If a patient is not taking a statin, it is reasonable to obtain a lipid profile at diabetes diagnosis, or at an initial medical evaluation, or every 5 years, or more often if indicated. Refer to ASCVD risk card for further guidance on initiating statin therapy.*
- *Recommendations for statin therapy should be made in addition to lifestyle therapy.*
- *Consider the following patients with diabetes mellitus (DM) to have similar risk to those with known CVD: men > age 40 with Type 2 + other coronary heart disease (CHD) risk factors OR age 50 with/without other CHD risk factors; women > 50 with Type 2 DM + other CHD risk factors OR age 55 with/without other CHD risk factors; men or women any age who have had DM for > 20 years with another risk factor OR men or women any age who have had DM > 25 years without another risk factor.*

Reference: Diabetes Care, Vol 39, S1:71.

Prepared by Jeanine P. Abrons, Molly Polzin, and Elisha Andreas

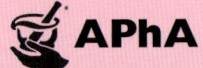

Cholesterol Management:
Use of Drug Classes Other than Statins

Results other than high LDL-C
Some patients with metabolic syndrome also may have low HDL-C or high triglycerides. The AHA/ACC guidelines for prevention of coronary artery disease recommend consideration of additional medications directed at these lipids such as niacin and fibrates.

When to consider use of nonstatins
May consider treatment with nonstatin medications in high-risk patients with the following clinical scenarios:
- Less than anticipated response to statins (after compliance has been confirmed)
- Inability to tolerate a less than recommended intensity of statin
- Complete intolerance to statin therapy
- Fibrates & omega-3 fatty acids may be considered in patients with persistent triglycerides > 500 mg/dL after lifestyle modifications & treatment of causes
- Complete intolerance to statin therapy
- Consider PCSK9 (-) as an adjunct to maximally tolerated statin therapy for treatment of HeFH or clinical ASCVD who needed greater ↓ of LDL-cholesterol

High-risk patients include
- Patients with clinical ASCVD
- Primary elevations of LDL-C > 190 mg/dL
- Patients with diabetes

Notes: LDL-C = low-density lipoprotein cholesterol; HDL-C = high-density lipoprotein cholesterol; PCSK9 = proprotein convertase subtilsin/kexin type 9; HeFH = heterozygous familial hypercholesterolemia; ASCVD = atherosclerotic cardiovascular disease.

Cholesterol Management:
Use of Drug Classes Other than Statins *(continued)*

Drug Classes Other Than Statins		
Drug Class	**Safety Considerations**	**Monitoring/Notes**
Bile Acid Sequestrants	**Do not use if** • Fasting triglycerides (TG) > 300 mg/dL • Type III hyperlipoproteinemia **Use cautiously in patients with** • Triglycerides 250 to 299 mg/dL **Discontinue use if** • TG increase to > 400 mg/dL	• Baseline: fasting lipid profile • Reevaluate 3 months after initiation and every 6 to 12 months thereafter
Cholesterol-Absorption Inhibitors (ezetimibe)	Discontinue with ALT (alanine aminotransferase) persistently > 3 times the upper limit of normal (ULN)	• Baseline: ALT/AST (aspartate transaminase) • When taken concomitantly with statins, monitor as clinically indicated • Monitor for CK ↑ associated with myopathy • May add with < 50% LDL-C ↓ while on high intensity statin • If TG > 300 mg/dL with use with statin, may add bile acid sequestrant
Fibrates	Gemfibrozil should not be used in conjunction with statins due to increased risk of muscle toxicities Fenofibrate may be considered in conjunction with low- or moderate-intensity statins	• Renal function should be evaluated prior to initiation of fibrate, within 3 months of initiation, and every 6 months thereafter • Do not initiate, and discontinue if estimated glomerular filtration rate (eGFR) is persistently < 30 mL/min/1.73 m² • If eGFR is 30 to 59 mL/min/1.73 m², dose of fenofibrate should not be higher than 54 mg • Limited LDL lowering action & randomized controlled trials (RCTs) do not support use in addition to statins
Niacin	**Do not use if or with** • ALT/AST ≥ 2 to 3 times ULN • Persistent, severe cutaneous reactions occur • Hyperglycemia • Acute gout • Gastrointestinal (GI) symptoms • New onset atrial fibrillation OR • Weight loss occurs **When to use** • May consider niacin as adjunct for ↓ TG. Not for use with high-dose statins and well-controlled LDL cholesterol	• Baseline: ALT/AST, fasting blood glucose or A1c, uric acid • Reevaluate during titration and every 6 months once maintenance dose is determined • Limited LDL lowering action & randomized controlled trials (RCTs) do not support use in addition to statins • In patients who develop cutaneous reactions: refer to guidelines • Reevaluate use in patients who develop other side effects
Omega-3 Fatty Acids	• Minimal safety considerations	• Evaluate for GI disturbances, skin changes, and bleeding • Assess TG prior to initiating • Monitor for ↑ in bleeding time
PCSK9 Inhibitors	• Common ADRs include injection site reactions, URIs, & nasopharyngitis • Require subcutaneous administration	• Baseline: fasting lipid panel • LDL-C: within 4 to 8 weeks of initiation or dose titration • Consider use in patients with very high risk & LDL-C ≥ 70 with statin therapy at max tolerated dose. ○ Use reasonable, but safety > 3 years is unknown/cost effectiveness if low.

Notes: CK = creatinine kinase; LDL = low-density lipoprotein; LDL-C = low-density lipoprotein cholesterol; ADR = adverse drug reaction; URI = upper respiratory infection.

Prepared by Nichole Bucci, Erica Maceira, Jeanine Abrons

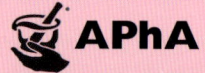

Direct Oral Anticoagulants

Medication/Consideration	Dabigatran (Pradaxa®) *Direct Thrombin Inhibitor (DTI)*	Rivaroxaban (Xarelto®) *Anti-Factor Xa Inhibitor*
FDA-Approved Indications *T = Treatment* *P = Prophylaxis*	• Stroke/emboli prevention in nonvalvular atrial fibrillation (NVAF)[T] • Deep vein thrombosis (DVT)/pulmonary embolism (PE) after 5 to 10 days of parenteral therapy[T] • ↓ DVT and PE recurrence in patients previously treated[P] • For DVT and PE prophylaxis in patients who have undergone hip replacement[P]	• Stroke/emboli prevention in NVAF[T] • DVT & PE[T] • DVT/PE risk ↓ after 6 months of prior treatment[P] • DVT/PE prophylaxis post-hip/knee replacement[P] • CAD prevention with or without aspirin: 2.5 mg BID

Usual Dosage

T = Treatment
P = Prophylaxis

Dabigatran (Pradaxa®)

Indication	T/P	Dose (Oral) – CrCl >30 mL/minute *After 5 to 10 days of parenteral therapy
NVAF	T	• 150 mg BID
DVT/PE	T P	• 150 mg BID • 150 mg BID after prior T
DVT/PE after hip replaced	P	• 110 mg on day 1, then 220 mg daily, start 1–4 hours after surgery/hemostasis achieved; for 28–35 days

Rivaroxaban (Xarelto®)

Indication	T/P	Dose (Oral)
NVAF	T	• 20 mg daily
DVT/PE	T P	• 15 mg BID x 21 days, then 20 mg daily • After 6 months of therapy: 10 mg daily per PI after prior T, with food
Post-Hip/Knee Prophylaxis	P	• Knee: 10 mg daily x 12 days • Hip: 10 mg daily x 35 days • CAD prevention with or without aspirin: 2.5 mg BID

Dose Adjustments

Based on creatinine clearance (CrCl)

Dabigatran (Pradaxa®)

Indication	T/P	Dose (Oral) – CrCl >30 mL/minute *After 5 to 10 days of parenteral therapy
NVAF	T	• At CrCl 15 to 30 mL/min: 75 mg BID • At CrCl <15 mL/min or dialysis: not recommended
DVT/PE	T	• At ≤ 30 mL/min: avoid use
DVT/PE after hip replaced	P	• At CrCl ≤30 mL/min or on dialysis: Dosing recommendations cannot be provided

Rivaroxaban (Xarelto®)

Indication	T/P	Dose (Oral)
NVAF	T	• At CrCl 15 to 50 mL/min: 15 mg daily • At CrCl <15mL/min: avoid use
Post-Hip/Knee Prophylaxis	T P	• At CrCl <30 mL/min: avoid use • At CrCl 30–50 mL/min: monitor for bleeding • Start 6–10 hours after surgery if adequate hemostasis with rivaroxaban for post-hip/knee prophylaxis

Significant Drug Interactions

Dabigatran (Pradaxa®)	Rivaroxaban (Xarelto®)
• Serious interactions & dose adjustments required with P-gp inducers/inhibitors; ketoconazole; dronedarone. See package insert for complete list.	• Serious interactions & dose adjustments required with P-gp inducers/inhibitors; cytochrome P450 3A4 inducers/inhibitors. See package insert.

Miscellaneous Considerations

Dabigatran (Pradaxa®)	Rivaroxaban (Xarelto®)
• Must administer capsule whole with full glass of water, do not break, chew, crush, or open • ESRD: Warfarin remains the drug of choice (DOC) per AHA/ACC • Cannot administer per tube	• Doses >10 mg MUST be taken with food; best with **evening meal if dosed once daily for NVAF** • ESRD: Warfarin remains the drug of choice (DOC) per AHA/ACC • Can be crushed

Notes: AHA = American Heart Association; ACC = American College of Cardiology; ESRD = end-stage renal disease; PI = package insert.

Direct Oral Anticoagulants *(continued)*

Medication/Consideration	Apixaban (Eliquis®) *Anti-Factor Xa Inhibitor*	Edoxaban (Savaysa®)
FDA-Approved Indications T = Treatment P = Prophylaxis	• Stroke/emboli prevention in nonvalvular atrial fibrillation (NVAF)[T] • Deep vein thrombosis (DVT)/pulmonary embolism (PE)[T] • DVT/PE risk ↓ after prior T • For DVT & PE prophylaxis in patients who have undergone hip replacement[P]	• Stroke/emboli prevention in NVAF[T]: **Contraindicated in CrCl > 95 mL/min due to ↑ risk of ischemic stroke compared to warfarin** • Not recommended for CrCl <15ml/min • DVT/PE treatment after 5–10 days of parenteral anticoagulant[T]

Usual Dosage
T = Treatment
P = Prophylaxis

^ Start 12 to 24 h after surgery

Apixaban (Eliquis®):

Indication	T/P	Dose (Oral)
NVAF	T	• 5 mg BID
DVT treatment	T P	• 10 mg BID for 7 days, then 5 mg BID • 2.5 mg BID after at least 6 months of T for DVT or PE
Post-Hip/Knee Prophylaxis^	P	• For Knee Replacement: 2.5 mg BID for 12 days • For Hip Replacement: 2.5 mg BID for 35 days

Edoxaban (Savaysa®):

Indication	T/P	Dose (Oral)
		*After 5 to 10 days of parenteral therapy
NVAF	T	• 60 mg daily **(contraindicated with CrCl > 95 mL/min due to ↑ risk of ischemic stroke compared to warfarin)**
DVT/PE	T	• 60 mg daily • Patient weight ≤ 60 kg or with P-gp inhibitors or with short-term use of macrolide antibiotics: 30 mg daily

Dose Adjustments
^ in dialysis may use dosing; weak evidence
Based on creatinine clearance (CrCl)

Apixaban (Eliquis®):

Indication	T/P	Dose (Oral) *Dose adjust in CrCl < 25 mL/min or SCR > 2.5 not studied
NVAF	T	• If patient has any 2 traits: age ≥ 80; weight ≤ 60 kg; serum creatinine (SCr) ≥ 1.5 mg/dL. THEN 2.5 mg BID
DVT/PE; Post Knee/Hip Prophylaxis^	P	• No dose adjustment for renal impairment for ESRD on dialysis; Use in CrCl < 15 ml/min not studied.

Edoxaban (Savaysa®):

Indication	T/P	Dose (Oral)
NVAF	T	• At CrCl 15 to 50 mL/min: 15 mg daily
DVT/PE	T	• At 15 to 50 mL/min or ≤ 60 kg who use certain P-gp inhibitors: 30 mg daily

Medication/Consideration	Apixaban (Eliquis®)	Edoxaban (Savaysa®)
Significant Drug Interactions	• Serious interactions & dose adjustments required with dual use of P-gp inducers/inhibitors; dual use of cytochrome P450 3A4 inducers/inhibitors. See package insert for complete list.	• Serious interactions & dose adjustments required with P-gp inhibitor in T of NVAF; for DVT/PE, ENGAGE AF-TIMI 48: dose ↓ led to ↓ levels compared to full dose T, DVT/PE no dose ↓ with concomitant use. See package insert for complete list.
Miscellaneous Considerations	• Can be taken with or without food • ESRD: Warfarin remains drug of choice (DOC) per AHA/ACC • Can be crushed • ESRD/HD approval based on case reports and case series; use caution & consider alternative	• Can be taken with or without food • No data on crushing &/or mixing/giving through feeding tubes • ESRD: Warfarin remains the drug of choice (DOC) per AHA/ACC

Notes: AHA = American Heart Association; ACC = American College of Cardiology; ESRD = end-stage renal disease; ESRD/HD = end-stage renal disease/hemodialysis; P-gp = P-glycoprotein.

Prepared by Apryl Jacobs, Erica Maceira, and Jeanine P. Abrons

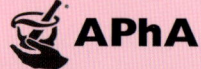

Injectable Anticoagulants

Injectable Anticoagulant/ Consideration	Unfractionated Heparin	Enoxaparin (Lovenox®)	Dalteparin (Fragmin®)	Fondaparinux (Arixtra®)
Dosing				
Prophylaxis	• 5000 units SC every 8 hours or 5000 units SC every 12 hours	• 30 mg SC every 12 hours OR 40 mg SC every 24 hours • Creatinine clearance (CrCl) < 30 mL/min: 30 mg SC every 24 hours • Do not use in dialysis	• 5000 units SC every 24 hours • Postsurgical prophylaxis for abdominal surgery: 2500 units SC every 24 hours • Postsurgical prophylaxis hip replacement: 2500 units 2 hours prior to surgery, then 2500 units 4 hours (or longer if failure to achieve hemostasis) after surgery, then 5000 units SC every 24 hours • Do not use in dialysis	• 2.5 mg SC every 24 hours • Do not use in patients with CrCl < 30 mL/min or patients < 50 kg
VTE Treatment	• SC: 333 units/kg SC once followed by 250 units/kg SC every 12 hours • IV: 80 units/kg or 5000 units IV bolus, then infusion of 18 units/kg (or 1000 units/hour) titrated to APTT or antifactor Xa assay (anti-Xa) • Goal: APTT = 1.5 to 2.5 x normal, anti-Xa = 0.3–0.7	• 1 mg/kg SC every 12 hours • 1.5 mg SC every 24 hours • CrCl < 30 mL/min: 1 mg/kg SC every 24 hours • Do not use in dialysis	• 100 units/kg SC every 12 hours OR • 200 units SC every 24 hours • Do not use in patients with CrCl < 30 mL/min	• < 50 kg: 5 mg SC every 24 hours • 50 to 100 kg: 7.5 mg SC every 24 hours • > 100 kg: 10 mg SC every 24 hours • Do not use in patients with CrCl < 30 mL/min
Half-life	• 1 to 2 hours • Impacted by obesity; renal function; malignancy; and presence of pulmonary embolism	• 5 to 7 hours • Impacted by renal function, pregnancy, obesity, and cumulative dose	• 2 to 5 hours • Impacted by renal function	• 17 to 21 hours • Impacted by renal function
Excretion	• Primarily hepatic but also by reticuloendothelial system • Higher dose: renal elimination may play more of a role	• Excretion: impacted by renal function, pregnancy, obesity, and cumulative dose	• Excretion: primarily renal (dose dependent)	• Excretion: urine (77% excreted unchanged)
Inhibited Factors	• Factors IIa, IXa, Xa, XIa, XIIa • Plasmin	• Factors Xa and IIa	• Factors Xa and IIa	• Factor Xa

Notes: All act through antithrombin III (so in patients with antithrombin III deficiency, these agents will predominantly be ineffective depending on the degree of deficiency). SC = subcutaneous; IV = intravenous; VTE = venous thromboembolism; APTT = activated partial thromboplastin time.

Prepared by: Erica Maceira, Nicole Bucci, and Shawn Phillips

Injectable Anticoagulants *(continued)*

Indications (X = Indicated)	Enoxaparin	Dalteparin	Fondaparinux
Deep vein thrombosis (DVT) prophylaxis in abdominal surgery	X	X	X
DVT prophylaxis in knee replacement surgery	X	------------------	X
DVT prophylaxis in hip replacement surgery	X	X	X (Hip fracture/replacement)
DVT prophylaxis in medical patients	X	X	------------------
Inpatient treatment of acute DVT with or without pulmonary embolism (PE)	X	------------------	X
Outpatient treatment of acute DVT without PE	X	------------------	X
Prophylaxis for unstable angina and non-Q-wave MI (myocardial infarction)	X	X	------------------
Treatment of acute STEMI managed medically or with subsequent PCI	X	------------------	------------------
Treatment of acute PE	------------------	------------------	X (with warfarin when initial treatment is administered in the hospital)
Cancer patients with acute DVT and/or PE	------------------	X	------------------

Notes: STEMI = ST-elevation myocardial infarction; PCI = percutaneous coronary intervention.

Prepared by Erica Maceira and Apryl Jacobs

Injectable Anticoagulants *(continued)*

Direct Thrombin Inhibitors (DTIs)

Injectable Anticoagulant/ Consideration	Argatroban	Bivalrudin (Angiomax®)
Indications	• Prophylaxis of coronary artery thrombosis in percutaneous coronary intervention patients with or at risk for HIT* • HIT treatment & prophylaxis*	• Anticoagulant use for patients undergoing PCI* • Management of HIT** • Off-label dosing also listed for ischemic heart and NSTEMI

Usual Dose	• Prophylaxis in PCI:
	  ○ 350 mcg/kg bolus over 3 min, then 35 mcg/kg/min IV continuous infusion
	  ○ Can re-bolus at 150 mcg/kg and/or ↑ rate to a maximum of 40 mcg/kg/min to achieve clotting time of 300–450 seconds
	• HIT treatment and prophylaxis:
	  ○ 2 mcg/kg/min continuous IV infusion; adjust until APTT is 1.5–3 times baseline to a maximum of 10 mcg/kg/min
		• During PCI for ACS:
		  ○ 0.75 mg/kg/bolus prior to procedure, followed by 1.75 mg/kg/hour for procedure duration; extended duration of infusion (up to 4 hours). Monitor ACT 5 min after bolus; give additional bolus of 0.3 mg/kg if needed.
		  ○ Bolus and infusion different if initiating prior to PCI.
		• Off label dosing for HIT:
		  ○ Data suggests dosing of 0.15 mg/kg/hour titrated to APTT 1.5–3 times control
		• Cardiac surgery in patients with acute/subacute HIT:
		  ○ Off-pump/on-pump dosing available

Dose Adjustments	• HIT treatment & prophylaxis with severe hepatic disease:
	  ○ Start at a rate of 0.5 mcg/kg/min
		• During PCI:
		  ○ No ↓ in bolus dose required for any degree of renal impairment
		  ○ CrCl < 30 mL/min: ↓ infusion rate to 1 mg/kg/hour
		  ○ ESRD on HD: ↓ infusion rate to 0.25 mg/kg/hour
		• Off label dosing for HIT:
		  ○ CrCl = 30–50 mL/min: 0.08 mg/kg/hour
		  ○ CrCl < 30 mL/min: 0.03 mg/kg/hour
		• Dialyzable: May require dose adjustments

Onset	• Immediate	• Immediate
Half-life	• 30 min to 1 hour • Increased in severe hepatic impairment to as high as 3 hours	• 25 min to 3.5 hours • Impacted by renal function
Excretion	• 25% renal; 16% unchanged • 65% fecal; 14% unchanged	• Excretion: Renal (dose dependent)
Inhibited Factors	• Factor II	• Factor II
Lab Interference	• When given with warfarin during bridging can falsely elevate INR due to lab interference	• PT/INR levels may ↑ in the absence of warfarin. If warfarin initiated, consider modification of initial PT/INR goals. • May need to consider modification of therapy depending on impact

Notes: * = FDA-approved indication; ** = off-label use. HIT = heparin-induced thrombocytopenia; SC = subcutaneous; IV = intravenous; PCI = percutaneous coronary intervention; ACS = acute coronary syndrome; ACT = activated clotting time; CrCl = creatinine clearance; ESRD = end-stage renal disease; HD = hemodialysis; APTT = activated partial thromboplast time; INR = international normalized ratio; PT = prothrombin time; NSTEMI = non-ST-elevation myocardial infarction.

Prepared by Erica Maceira, Shawn Phillips, Nicole Bucci

Perioperative Management of Direct Oral Anticoagulants

Medication/ Renal Function (Creatinine Clearance [CrCl])	Half Life (T ½)	Low Bleeding Risk Surgery: Timing of Last Dose	High Bleeding Risk Surgery: Timing of Last Dose	When to Resume Therapy	
				LOW Bleeding Risk Surgery	HIGH Bleeding Risk Surgery
Dabigatran (Pradaxa®)					
> 50 mL/min	T½ = 12–17 hours; 14–17 hours in elderly	2 days before procedure	3 days before procedure	Resume on the day after procedure (24 hours postoperative)	Resume 2–3 days after procedure (48–72 hours postoperative)
30–50 mL/min	T½ = 15–18 hours	3 days before procedure	4–5 days before procedure	Resume on the day after procedure (24 hours postoperative)	Resume 2–3 days after procedure (48–72 hours postoperative)
Rivaroxaban (Xarelto®)					
> 30 mL/min	T½ = 5–9 hours	2 days before procedure	3 days before procedure	Resume on the day after procedure (24 hours postoperative)	Resume 2–3 days after procedure (48–72 hours postoperative)
< 30 mL/min	T½ = 9–10 hours	Varies based on patient/ procedure	Varies based on patient/ procedure	Resume on the day after procedure (24 hours postoperative)	Resume 2–3 days after procedure (48–72 hours postoperative)
Apixaban (Eliquis®)					
> 30 mL/min	T½ = 12–18 hours	Varies based on patient/ procedure	Varies based on patient/ procedure	Resume on the day after procedure (24 hours postoperative)	Resume 2–3 days after procedure (48–72 hours postoperative)
< 30 mL/min	T½ = ~ 17 hours	2 days before procedure	3 days before procedure	Resume on the day after procedure (24 hours postoperative)	Resume 2–3 days after procedure (48–72 hours postoperative)
Edoxaban (Savaysa®)					
> 50 mL/min	T½ = 10–14 hours	2 days before procedure	3 days before procedure	Resume on the day after procedure (24 hours postoperative)	Resume 2–3 days after procedure (48–72 hours postoperative)

Note: For patients at high risk for thromboembolism and bleed risk after surgery, consider administering a reduced dose of dabigatran (75 mg BID), rivaroxaban (10 mg daily), or apixaban (2.5 mg BID) on the evening after surgery and on the first postoperative day.

These recommendations are for patients not undergoing neuraxial procedures. For patients undergoing neuraxial procedures, see the American Society of Regional Anesthesia & Pain Medicine guidelines: https://journals.lww.com/rapm/Fulltext/2015/05000/Interventional_Spine_and_Pain_Procedures_in.2.aspx (Accessed 2018).

Reference: Doherty J, Gluckman T, Hucker W, et al. 2017 ACC Expert Consensus Decision Pathway for Periprocedural Management of Anticoagulation in Patients With Nonvalvular Atrial Fibrillation: A Report of the American College of Cardiology Clinical Expert Consensus Document Task Force. J Am Coll Cardiol. 2017 Feb 21;69(7);871-898.

Prepared by Erica Maceria and Apryl Jacobs

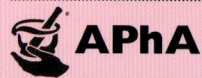

Common Warfarin Drug Interactions

Drug Class or Medication That Interacts with Warfarin	Impact on Warfarin levels: Potential Management		
Antibiotics E.g., ciprofloxacin; clarithromycin; erythromycin; metronidazole; sulfamethoxazole/trimethoprim	Majority ↑		
	Metronidazole: ↑; consider alternatives. If used together, consider ↓ warfarin dose by 25–50%	**Dicloxacillin:** ↓; more significant if course >14 days	
	Rifampin: ↓; may consider ↑ of warfarin dose by 25–50%.	**Ciprofloxacin:** ↑ At 2–5 days; may consider ↓ warfarin dose by 10–15%	
	Clarithromycin: At 3–7 days; may ↓ dose warfarin 15–25%	**Erythromycin:** At 3–5 days; may consider ↓ warfarin dose by 10–15%	
	Sulfamethoxazole/Trimethoprim: ↑ At 2–5 days; may consider ↓ warfarin dose by 25–40%		
Antifungal Medications: E.g., fluconzole; miconazole	↑; At 2–3 days; consider initial dose ↓ by 25–30%; may need to ↓ up to 80% with fluconazole		
Antidepressants: E.g., quetiapine; SSRIs; tramadol	↑; **Tramadol:** Warfarin dose may need to be ↓ by 25–30%		
Antiplatelet Medications	Does not increase INR, just ↑ bleeding risk. Monitor for signs/symptoms.		
Anticoagulant Medications	Does not increase INR, just ↑ bleeding risk. Monitor for signs/symptoms.		
Amiodarone	↑; slow ↑ over time (e.g., 6–8 weeks); empiric warfarin dose by 10–25% at week 1; may ↓ warfarin dose by 25–60% eventually		
Acetaminophen	↑; with high doses (limited dose to < 2000 mg/day → avoid use of higher doses if possible); onset at 2–5 days		
Carbamazepine	↓; warfarin dose may need to be ↑ by 50–100%; ↓ warfarin dose by 50% when stopping		
Fenofibrate	↑; warfarin dose may need to be ↑ by 50–100%; ↓ warfarin dose by 50% when stopping		
Gemfibrozil	↑; may ↓ dose warfarin by 10–15%		
Phenobarbital	↓; warfarin dose may need to be ↑ by 30–60%		
Rosuvastatin	↑; may ↓ dose warfarin by 10–25%		
	↑ Levels		↓ Levels
Alternative Therapies Note: Please refer to additional reference for more extensive list	C: cannabis; capsicum; chamomile; clove; cranberry G: garlic; ginger; gingko; grapefruit		G: ginseng; green tea; goldenseal Other: noni; parsley; St. John's wort; yarrow

Notes: For all significant drug interactions, monitor international normalized ratio (INR) more often.

This table is not all inclusive; it provides a guidance for recall of common interactions that require dose adjustment of warfarin; e.g., anti-inflammatory & antiplatelet medications should have increased monitoring for signs & symptoms of bleeding; SSRI = selective serotonin reuptake inhibitor.

Sample References: http://www.ncbi.nlm.nih/pmc/articles/PMC1942100/pdf/2007081 4s00018p369.pdf (Accessed 2018); Alternative Therapies Reference: National Center for Complementary and Alternative Medicine (http://nccam.nih.gov/health/herbsataglance.html (Accessed 2018).

Prepared by Jeannie P. Abrons and Erica Maceira.

Warfarin Dosing According to the 9th Edition of CHEST Guidelines

Monitoring Based on CHEST Guidelines

- In hospitalized patients, INR monitoring is typically performed daily until therapeutic range is achieved and maintained for at least 2 consecutive days.
- In an outpatient setting, INRs will be monitored more frequently initially (e.g., every 1 to 3 days) and then frequency between INRs can be increased once a stable dose is achieved.
- For outpatient with consistently stable INRs, testing frequency may be extended up to 12 weeks (rather than every 4 weeks).
- Optimal frequency of monitoring may be impacted by patient compliance, comorbid conditions, medication use or adherence, and dose response.
- It is important to know the reason for being on warfarin as this will impact the duration of therapy.

Consider influence of factors that may be associated with higher risk of bleeding

- Advanced age
- Serious comorbid conditions (cancer; renal use or insufficiency; liver disease; arterial hypertension; prior stroke; alcohol abuse; other therapies)

If fluctuations occur—consider the reasons for the fluctuation

- Inaccuracy of INR testing
- Changes in dietary vitamin K intake
- Changes in absorption/distribution/metabolism/excretion of vitamin K or warfarin
- Concomitant medical conditions

Management of Out-of-Range INRs Based on CHEST Guidelines

- For previously stable patients with a single out-of-range INR of ≤ 0.5 below or above the therapeutic range, the current dose may be continued and testing can be done within 1 to 2 weeks.
- Risk to patient is considered to be low.
- For stable patients with single subtherapeutic INR, do not routinely bridge with a parenteral anticoagulant.
- With major bleeding, rapid reversal of anticoagulation with four-factor prothrombin complex concentrate is suggested rather than with plasma.
- Add vitamin K 5 to 10 mg oral or intravenous (IV) injection rather than reversal with coagulation factors alone.

Sample INR Level and Corresponding Evidence of Bleeding:

INR Level and Evidence of Bleeding	Recommendation
4.5 to 10 and No Evidence of Bleeding	Routine use of vitamin K not recommended
Greater than 10 and No Evidence of Bleeding	Administer oral vitamin K
Evidence of Bleeding	Kcentra® and vitamin K

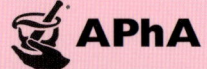

Warfarin Dosing According to the 9th Edition of CHEST Guidelines *(continued)*

Target INRs
- The CHEST 9th Edition Guidelines recommend therapeutic INRs of 2 to 3 rather than lower (< 2) or higher (3 to 5) ranges for most indications (Grade 1B).
- Higher intensity INR ranges exist for patients with mechanical mitral valves or with mechanical aortic valve and other risk factors.

Initiation of Warfarin Dosing Based on CHEST Guidelines
- CHEST 9th Edition Guidelines suggest patients sufficiently healthy to be treated as outpatients may start at 10 mg for 2 days followed by dosing based on INR.
- In patients with acute thromboembolism, therapy may be started on day 1 or 2 of an injectable anticoagulant rather than waiting to start.
- Many patients will be started at doses between 5 and 10 mg.
- Examples of when to consider a starting dose of < 5 mg:

• Elderly	• Impaired nutrition
• Liver disease	• High bleeding risk
• Congestive heart failure	

- 2 to 3 mg initial dose appropriate for patient with heart valve replacement.

Counseling Points Related to Warfarin
- Many drug interactions exist. Instruct the patient about the likelihood of a drug interaction and to report all medication changes.
- Know the reason that warfarin is being prescribed, as this will impact the duration of therapy.

Consistency is key with

• Medication adherence	• INR monitoring
• Medication interactions	• Vitamin K intake

Ask questions if recent changes have occurred:

• Does the new med interact?	• Has there been recent illness?
• Have there been dietary changes?	• How does patient take medication (assess adherence)?

Signs and symptoms of bleeding
- Stress the importance of reporting signs or symptoms to the doctor and pharmacist.
- This may mean that warfarin is dosed at too high a level or that further monitoring is needed.

Warfarin Strengths and Colors

1 mg:	2 mg:	2.5 mg:	3 mg:	4 mg:	5 mg:	6 mg:	7.5 mg:	10 mg:
Pink	Purple	Green	Brown	Blue	Orange	Teal	Yellow	White

Other Warfarin Resources (Accessed November 2018)

- http://www.warfarindosing.org
- http://www.coumadin.bmscustomerconnect.com

Prepared by Jeanine P. Abrons

Alterations to Warfarin Dose Maintenance Therapy

This flowchart does not replace the need for clinical decision making. Decisions regarding patient care should be made in accordance with clinical judgment. Care should be given as medically necessary in the patient's best interest based upon independent clinical reasoning, clinician judgment, and objective data. Percentage adjustments may vary by institutional nomogram as well (e.g., INR < 2, increase by 10 to 15%; INR 3.1 to 3.5, decrease by 0 to 10%). This card was created by referencing multiple nomograms.

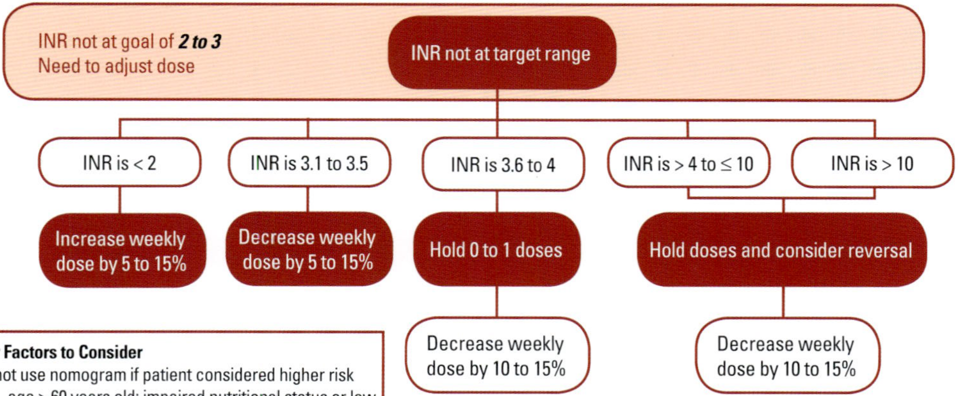

INR not at goal of *2 to 3*
Need to adjust dose

- INR is < 2 → **Increase weekly dose by 5 to 15%**
- INR is 3.1 to 3.5 → **Decrease weekly dose by 5 to 15%**

INR not at target range

- INR is 3.6 to 4 → **Hold 0 to 1 doses** → Decrease weekly dose by 10 to 15%
- INR is > 4 to ≤ 10 / INR is > 10 → **Hold doses and consider reversal** → Decrease weekly dose by 10 to 15%

Other Factors to Consider
- Do not use nomogram if patient considered higher risk (e.g., age > 60 years old; impaired nutritional status or low body mass index [BMI]; liver disease [Child-Pugh Grade B/C]; taking medications known to increase warfarin activity or bleeding risk; recent major surgery or high bleeding risk)
- Setting (inpatient or outpatient)
- Frequency of monitoring possible
- Recheck INRs after any alterations (time varies)

Parameters That May Impact INRs
- Patient nonadherence (missing/ extra doses)
- Alcohol use
- Changes in health (fever, diarrhea/nausea/vomiting)
- Changes in vitamin K intake
- Medication changes
- Bleeding or thromboembolism

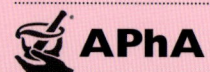

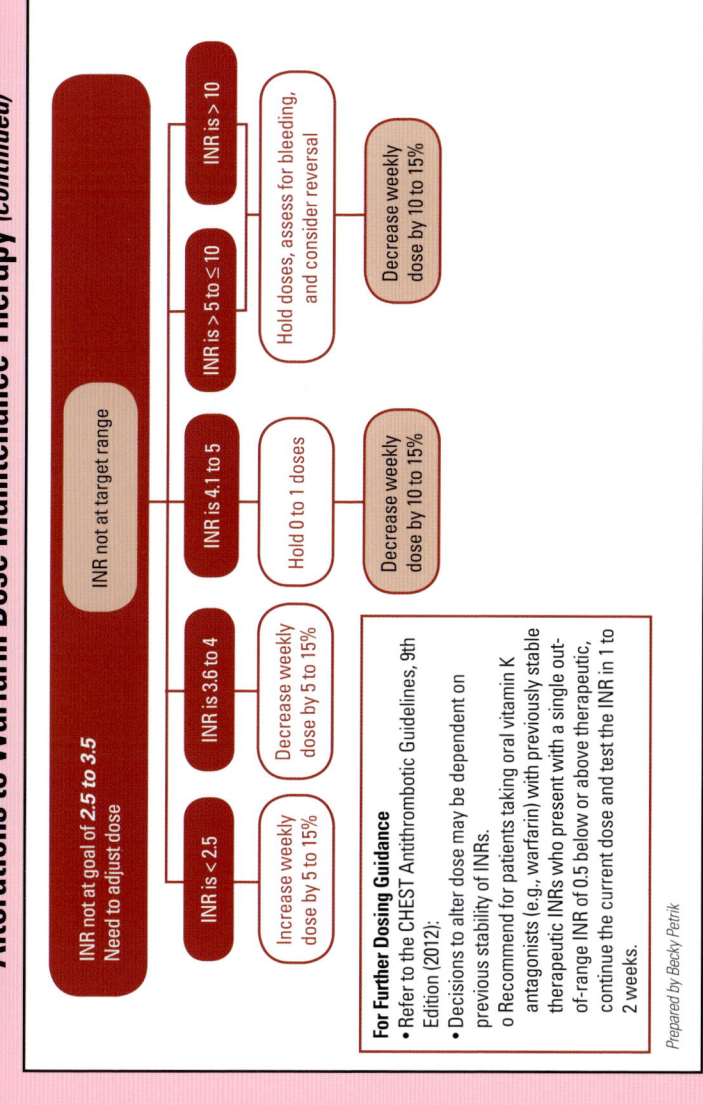

INR not at goal of *2.5 to 3.5*
Need to adjust dose

INR not at target range

- **INR is < 2.5**
  - Increase weekly dose by 5 to 15%

- **INR is 3.6 to 4**
  - Decrease weekly dose by 5 to 15%

- **INR is 4.1 to 5**
  - Hold 0 to 1 doses
  - Decrease weekly dose by 10 to 15%

- **INR is > 5 to ≤ 10**
  - Hold doses, assess for bleeding, and consider reversal
  - Decrease weekly dose by 10 to 15%

- **INR is > 10**

For Further Dosing Guidance
- Refer to the CHEST Antithrombotic Guidelines, 9th Edition (2012):
- Decisions to alter dose may be dependent on previous stability of INRs.
  - o Recommend for patients taking oral vitamin K antagonists (e.g., warfarin) with previously stable therapeutic INRs who present with a single out-of-range INR of 0.5 below or above therapeutic, continue the current dose and test the INR in 1 to 2 weeks.

Prepared by Becky Petrik

Diabetes Treatment Guidelines

For more comprehensive information about current approaches to the diagnosis and treatment of diabetes, visit the American Diabetes Association Standards of Medical Care—2019 website at *https://professional.diabetes.org/content-page/standards-medical-care-diabetes (Accessed 2019).*

Criteria for Diagnosis of Diabetes

Diagnostic Tool	Value Associated with Diagnosis of Diabetes
Fasting Plasma Glucose (FPG)[a]	≥ 126 mg/dL • In absence of unequivocal hyperglycemia, diagnosis requires two abnormal test results from the same sample or two separate samples
Random Plasma Glucose	≥ 200 mg/dL with symptoms (polyuria; polydipsia; unexplained weight loss) • Value measured without regard to last meal • Only diagnostic with classic symptoms of hyperglycemia or hyperglycemic crisis
Oral Glucose Tolerance Test	≥ 200 mg/dL 2 hours post 75 g glucose challenge • In absence of unequivocal hyperglycemia, diagnosis requires two abnormal test results from the same sample or two separate samples
Hemoglobin A1c[b]	≥ 6.5% • Performed in a laboratory using a method that is NGSP certified[c] and standardized to the DCCT assay[d]

a: Fasting is defined as no caloric intake for at least 8 hours.

b: In conditions associated with ↑ red blood cell turnover (e.g., sickle cell disease, pregnancy [2nd & 3rd trimester], hemodialysis, recent blood loss/transfusion, or erythropoietin therapy): Only plasma blood glucose should be used to diagnose diabetes.

c: National Glycohemoglobin Standardization Program.

d: Diabetes Control and Complications Trial.

Practitioner may select one diagnostic tool above and in absence of unequivocal hyperglycemia should confirm results with repeat testing.

Criteria Associated with Increased Risk for Diabetes

Diagnostic Tool	Value Associated with Diagnosis of Diabetes
Impaired Fasting Glucose[a]	100 to 125 mg/dL
Impaired Glucose Tolerance	140 to 199 mg/dL • 2 hours post 75 g glucose challenge
Hemoglobin A1c	Range of 5.7% to 6.4%

a: Fasting is defined as no caloric intake for at least 8 hours.

Note: Patients age 45 years old, with body mass index (BMI) > 25 kg/m² or > 23 kg/m² in Asian Americans, and/or adults with ≥ 1 risk factor, even if asymptomatic, should be screened for diabetes with the above diagnostic tools and criteria. Risk factors include first-degree relative with diabetes; high-risk race/ethnicity (e.g., African American, Latino, Native American, Asian American, Pacific Islander); history of cardiovascular disease; hypertension (> 140/90 mmHg or on therapy for hypertension); HDL ≥ 35 mg/dL and/or a triglyceride level ≥ 250 mg/dL; women with polycystic ovarian syndrome; physical inactivity; other clinical conditions associated with insulin resistance (e.g., severe obesity, acanthosis nigricans). For all patients, testing should be initiated at age 45 and offered at 3-year intervals. In patients with prediabetes or increased risk for diabetes, testing should be done more frequently (yearly).

Updated by Jeanine P. Abrons, Elisha Andreas, and Molly Polzin.

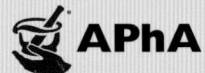

Goals of Care for Patients with Diabetes

Area of Care	Description of Care
Assess key patient characteristics	• Current lifestyle • Comorbidities • Clinical characteristics (e.g., age, hemoglobin A1c, weight) • Issues such as motivation and depression • Cultural and socioeconomic context
Consider specific factors that impact the choice of treatment	• Individualized hemoglobin A1c target • Impact on weight and hypoglycemia • Side effect profile of medication • Complexity of regimen (e.g., frequency, mode of administration) • A regimen that optimizes adherence and persistence • Access, cost, and availability of medication
Create a management plan with shared decision making	• Involves an educated and informed patient or family caregiver • Seeks patient preferences • Empowers the patient • Effective consultation with motivational interviewing, goal setting, and shared decision making
Agree on the management plan	• Specific SMART goals (Specific; Measurable; Achievable; Realistic; Time limited)
Implement the management plan	• Patients not meeting goals generally should be seen at least every 3 months if progress is being made; more frequent initial contact is desirable
Provide ongoing monitoring and support to evaluate the following	• Emotional well-being • Tolerability of medication • Glycemic status • Biofeedback (e.g., self-monitoring of blood glucose, weight, step count, hemoglobin A1c, blood pressure, and lipids)
Review and agree on a management plan	• Review management plan • Mutually agree on changes • Ensure the modification of therapy is implemented • Undertake a decision cycle regularly (at least once or twice a year)

American Diabetes Association. Standards of Medical Care in Diabetes—2019. Diabetes Care. 2019;42(suppl 1):S1-S193.

Prepared by Jeanine Abrons and Elisha Andreas

Associated Goals for Adults with Diabetes

Associated Goals	Value of Goal
Glycemic Control (A1c)[a]	ADA*: < 8 for patients at risk for severe hypoglycemia or < 7%[b] AACE**: < 6.5%[c]
Preprandial Capillary Plasma Glucose	ADA: 80 to 130 mg/dL[b] AACE: < 110 mg/dL
Postprandial Capillary Plasma Glucose	ADA: < 180 mg/dL[b,d] AACE: < 140 mg/dL
Blood Pressure (Systolic)	ADA: < 140 mmHg[e] AACE: < 130 mmHg[f]
Blood Pressure (Diastolic)	ADA: < 90 mmHg AACE: < 80 mmHg

*Notes: *American Diabetes Association (ADA) Standards of Medical Care 2018; **American Association of Clinical Endocrinologists (AACE) and American College of Endocrinology Comprehensive Type 2 Diabetes Management Algorithm 2018.*

a: Perform A1c testing at least 2 times per year in patients meeting treatment goals (and who have stable glycemic control). Perform A1c testing quarterly in patients with changes to therapy or who are not meeting glycemic goals.

b: More or less stringent glycemic goals may be appropriate for individual patients. Goal of < 8% may be considered in patients with increased risk of hypoglycemia, limited life expectancy, advanced microvascular or macrovascular complications, extensive co-morbid conditions, or long-standing diabetes in whom goals are difficult to achieve despite self-management education, appropriate monitoring, and effective dosing of therapies. Goal of < 6.5% may be considered for patients with short duration of diabetes, type 2 diabetes treated with lifestyle interventions or metformin only, long-life expectancy, or no significant cardiovascular disease.

c: For patients without concurrent serious illness and at low hypoglycemic risk; level ≥ 6.5% for patients with concurrent illness and at risk for hypoglycemia. A1c targets must be individualized.

d: Postprandial glucose may be targeted if A1c goals are not met despite reaching preprandial glucose goals. Measurements should be made 1–2 hours after the beginning of a meal, generally represents peak levels.

e: Lower systolic (< 130 mmHg) and diastolic (< 80 mmHg) blood pressure goals may be considered with diabetes and hypertension in patients with higher cardiovascular risk (e.g., existing atherosclerotic cardiovascular disease > 15%) if tolerated.

f: Less stringent goals may be considered for frail patients with complicated comorbidities or those who have adverse medication effects. More intensive goal (e.g., < 120/80 mmHg) should be considered for patients if this goal can be safely reached without adverse medication-related effects.

Updated by Jeanine P. Abrons, Molly Polzin and Elisha Andreas.

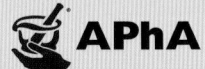

Insulin and Insulin Analogues

Type	Generic Name (Trade Name)	Onset (hours)	Peak (hours)	Duration (hours)	Administration Route
Ultra Rapid Acting					
Analogue	**Asprart** (Fiasp®)	0.04	1 to 1.5	5	Subcutaneous (SC) injection
Rapid Acting					
Analogue	Aspart (Novolog®)	0.2 to 0.3	1 to 3	3 to ≤ 5	SC [Injection/CSII]
	Glulisine (Apidra®)	0.2 to 0.5	1.6 to 2.8		
	Lispro (Humalog®, Admelog®)	< 0.25	0.5 to 2.5		
Short Acting					
Human	Regular (Humulin R®, Novolin®)	0.5	2.5 to 5	4 to 12	Daily maintenance use: SC [Injection/CSII]; continuous infusion may be used in other instances
	Regular U-500 (Humulin R® Concentrated)			Up to 24	SC [Injection/CSII]
Intermediate Acting					
Human	NPH (Humulin-N®, Novolin-N®)	1 to 2	9 to 12	14 to 24	SC
Long Acting					
Analogue; Human	Degludec (Tresiba®)	~ 1	Not applicable	Not applicable	SC
	Detemir (Levemir®)	3 to 4	3 to 9	6 to 23	
	Glargine (Lantus®)		Not applicable	10.8 to > 24	
	Glargine (Basaglar®)			≥ 24	
	Glargine (Toujeo®)	6			
Insulin Combinations					
Combination	Degludec + Aspart (Ryzodeg® 70/30)	0.23	Not applicable	> 24	SC
	NPH + Regular (Humulin® 70/30; Novolin® 70/30)	0.5	2 to 12	18 to 24	
	Lispro protamine + Lispro (Humalog® Mix 50/50; Humalog® Mix 75/25)	0.25 to 0.5	50/50 Mix: 0.8 to 48 75/25 Mix: 1 to 6.5	14 to 24	
	Aspart protamine + Aspart (Novolog® Mix 70/30)	0.2 to 0.3	1 to 4	18 to 24	
	Glargine + GLP-1 Agonist (Soliqua® 100/33)	Not listed	2.5 to 3	$T \frac{1}{2}$ = 3 h; Clearance = 35 L/h	
	Degludec + GLP-1 Agonist (Xultophy® 100/3.6)		Not applicable	> 24 (see individual drugs)	

Note: CSII = continuous subcutaneous insulin infusion; GLP = glucagon-like peptide.

Updated by Jasmine Mangrum and Jeanine P. Abrons

Management of Type 2 Diabetes

Therapeutic Approach	When to Use	When to Consider Next Approach	Other Notes
1. Monotherapy	• Use as an initial approach except when A1c ≥ 9% **Consideration Area / Specifics to Drug/Approach** Efficacy • High Hypoglycemia risk • Low Associated weight impact • Neutral/loss Notable side effects • Gastrointestinal (GI)/lactic acidosis Costs • Low	• If A1c goal not achieved after ~ 3 months with treatment approach: proceed to use of 2-drug combination (dual therapy)	• Use with lifestyle management
2. Dual Therapy (metformin + additional medication)	• Consider as an initial approach when A1c ≥ 9% or in patients with newly diagnosed type 2 diabetes who have A1c ≥ 1.5% above their glycemic target.	• If A1c goal not achieved after ~ 3 months with treatment approach: proceed to use of 3-drug combination (triple therapy)	• Choice of additional medication dependent upon patient/disease-specific factors • Use with lifestyle management

Consideration Area table (Monotherapy):

Consideration Area	Specifics to Drug/Approach
Efficacy	• High
Hypoglycemia risk	• Low
Associated weight impact	• Neutral/loss
Notable side effects	• Gastrointestinal (GI)/lactic acidosis
Costs	• Low

Dual Therapy drug class table:

Drug Class	Efficacy	Hypoglycemia Risk	Associated Weight Impact	Notable Side Effects	Costs
Sulfonylureas	High	Moderate	Gain	Hypoglycemia	Low
Thiazolidinediones	High	Low	Gain	Edema, HF	Low
DPP-4 inhibitors	Intermediate	Low	Neutral	Rare	High
SGLT2 inhibitors	Intermediate	Low	Loss	GU, dehydration	High
GLP-1 receptor agonist	High	Low	Loss	GI	High
Insulin (basal)	Highest	High	Gain	Hypoglycemia	High

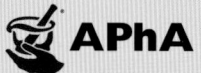

26

Management of Type 2 Diabetes *(continued)*

Therapeutic Approach	When to Use	When to Consider Next Approach	Other Notes
3. Triple Therapy (metformin + 2 additional medications)	• Consider	• If A1c goal not achieved after ~ 3 months with treatment approach * patient (1) on oral combo, move to insulin (basal) or GLP-1-RA, (2) on GLP-1-RA + insulin (basal), or (3) on optimal insulin (basal) + GLP-1-RA or mealtime insulin • Maintain metformin with change while other oral agents may be DC'd	• Choice of additional medication dependent upon patient/disease-specific factors • Use with lifestyle management

When to Use (Triple Therapy combinations):

Sulfonylurea +	Thiazolidinediones +	DPP-4 Inhibitor +	SGLT2 Inhibitors +	GLP-1 Receptor Agonist +	Insulin (Basal) +
SU	SU	SU	SU	SU	TZD
May select any 1 agent below to use in combination with 1st row					
DPP-4-I	DPP-4-I	TZD	TZD	TZD	DPP-4-I
SGLT2-I	SGLT2-I	SGLT2-I	DPP-4-I	SGLT2-I	SGLT2-I
GLP-1-RA	GLP-1-RA	Insulin	GLP-1-RA	Insulin	GLP-1-RA
Insulin	Insulin		Insulin		

Combination
• Consider as an initial approach with A1c ≥ 10%, blood glucose ≥ 300 mg/dL OR patient is markedly symptomatic

Notes: HF = heart failure; GU = genitourinary; TZD = thiazolidinediones; DPP-4-I = DPP-4 inhibitors; SGLT2-I = SGLT2 inhibitors; GLP-1—RA = GLP-1 receptor agonist; SU = sulfonylureas; DC'd = discontinued; HF = heart failure; GU = genitourinary; GI = gastrointestinal.

Prepared by Jeanine Abrons

Injectable Type 2 Diabetes Medications

Drug Class	Generic Name/Brand Name	Usual Starting Dose	Maximum Daily Dose	Notable Side Effects	Special Considerations/Notes
GLP-1 AGONISTS	**Exenatide** (Byetta®)	5 mcg twice daily	10 mcg twice daily	• Headache • Hypoglycemia • Nausea • Diarrhea • Injection site reaction	• Administer 60 minutes prior to a meal • Subcutaneous administration • Box warning: risk of developing thyroid C-cell tumors
	Exenatide Extended Release (Bydureon®)	2 mg once weekly	Not applicable	• Headache • Hypoglycemia • Nausea • Diarrhea • Injection site nodule	• Subcutaneous administration • Box warning: risk of developing thyroid C-cell tumors • Use right away after mixing • Take with or without food
	Albiglutide (Tanzeum®)	30 mg once weekly	50 mg once weekly	• Hypoglycemia • Diarrhea • Injection site reactions	• Subcutaneous administration • Box warning: risk of developing thyroid C-cell tumors • Take with or without food
	Dulaglutide (Trulicity®)	0.75 mg once weekly	1.5 mg once weekly	• Nausea • Diarrhea • Vomiting	• Subcutaneous administration • Box warning: risk of developing thyroid C-cell tumors • Take with or without food
	Liraglutide (Victoza®)	See Special Consideration/Notes	1.8 mg once daily	• Tachycardia • Headache • Hypoglycemia • Nausea • Constipation • Vomiting	• 0.6 mg once daily for 1 week, then increase to 1.2 mg once daily; may increase up to 1.8 mg once daily if optimal glycemic response not achieved with 1.2 mg once daily • Initial starting dose is intended to reduce gastrointestinal (GI) symptoms and does not provide effective glycemic control • Subcutaneous administration • Box warning: risk of developing thyroid C-cell tumors • Take with or without food • Drink noncaffeine liquids

Prepared by Jasmine Mangrum and Jeanine P. Abrons.

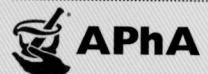

Initiating Therapy in Children with Intermittent Asthma Severity

Consideration	Initiating Therapy in Children with Intermittent Asthma Severity	
	Ages 0 to 4	Ages 5 to 11
Symptom frequency	≤ 2 days/week	≤ 2 days/week
Number of nighttime awakenings	0	2 times per month
Frequency of use of SABA to control symptoms	≤ 2 days/week	≤ 2 days/week
Extent of limitation of normal activity	No limitation	No limitation
Lung Function • Predicted FEV_1 or personal best peak flow • FEV_1/FVC	N/A	Normal FEV_1 between exacerbations • > 80% • > 85%
Exacerbations that require oral systemic corticosteroids Considerations: severity/interval since last exacerbation	0 to 1 time per year	0 to 1 time per year
Recommended Step Therapy Should not replace clinical decision making & individual patient needs	Step 1: • Reevaluate in 2 to 6 weeks: level of asthma control • If no clear benefit in 4 to 6 weeks: stop treatment & consider another diagnosis	Step 1: • Reevaluate in 2 to 6 weeks: level of asthma control • Adjust therapy accordingly

Note: SABA = short-acting beta-agonists; FEV_1 = forced expiratory volume in one second; FVC = forced vital capacity; N/A = not applicable.

References: Based on Figure 4-2a, Classifying Asthma Severity & Initiating Therapy in Children 0 to 4 Years of Age; Figure 4-2b, Classifying Asthma Severity & Initiating Treatment in Children 5 to 11 Years of Age from the National Asthma Education & Prevention Program Expert Panel Report III: Guidelines for the Diagnosis & Management of Asthma. Bethesda, MD: National Heart, Lung, and Blood Institute, 2007. www.nhlbi.nih.gov/guidelines/asthma/asthgdln.htm (Accessed November 2018); Global Strategy for Asthma Management & Prevention, Global Initiative for Asthma (GINA) also may be referenced. http://ginasthma.org/gina-reports/ (Accessed November 2018).

Prepared by Jeanine P. Abrons

Initiating Therapy in Children with Persistent Asthma Severity

Consideration	Initiating Therapy in Children with Persistent Asthma Severity					
	Ages 0 to 4			Ages 5 to 11		
	Mild	Moderate	Severe	Mild	Moderate	Severe
Symptom frequency	> 2 days/week, but not daily	Daily	Throughout the day	> 2 days/week, but not daily	Daily	Throughout the day
Number of nighttime awakenings	1 to 2 times per month	3 to 4 times per month	> 1 time per week	3 to 4 times per month	> 1 time per week, but not nightly	Often; 7 times per week
Frequency of use of SABA to control symptoms	> 2 days/week, but not daily	Daily	Several times per day	> 2 days/week, but not daily	Daily	Several times/day
Extent of limitation of normal activity	Minor	Some	Extreme	Minor	Some	Extreme
Lung Function • Predicted FEV, or personal best peak flow • FEV$_1$/FVC	N/A	N/A	N/A	• > 80% • > 80%	• 60 to 80% • 75 to 80%	• < 60% • < 75%
Exacerbations that require oral systemic corticosteroids Considerations: severity/interval since last exacerbation	≥ 2 in 6 months OR > 4 wheezing episodes/year lasting > 1 day & persistent asthma risk factors			≥ 2 times per year Relative annual risk may be related to FEV$_1$		
Recommended Step Therapy Should not replace clinical decision making & individual patient needs	Step 2	Step 3 & consider short course of oral systemic corticosteroid		Step 2	Step 3: medium-dose ICS OR Step 4 and consider short course of oral systemic corticosteroids	

Note: SABA = short-acting beta-agonists; FEV$_1$ = forced expiratory volume in one second; FVC = forced vital capacity; ICS = inhaled corticosteroid; N/A = not applicable.

References: Based on Figure 4-2a, Classifying Asthma Severity & Initiating Therapy in Children 0 to 4 Years of Age; Figure 4-2b, Classifying Asthma Severity & Initiating Treatment in Children 5 to 11 Years of Age from the National Asthma Education & Prevention Program Expert Panel Report III: Guidelines for the Diagnosis & Management of Asthma. Bethesda, MD: National Heart, Lung, and Blood Institute, 2007. www.nhlbi.nih.gov/guidelines/asthma/asthgdln.htm (Accessed November 2018). Global Strategy for Asthma Management & Prevention, Global Initiative for Asthma (GINA) also may be referenced. http://ginasthma.org/gina-reports/ (Accessed November 2018).

Prepared by Jeanine P. Abrons

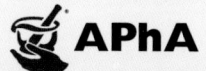

Adjusting Asthma Therapy in Children Ages 0 to 4

Consideration	Asthma Control and Therapy Adjustment (based on most impairment, risk, and recall of previous 2 to 4 weeks)		
	Well Controlled	**Not Well Controlled**	**Very Poorly Controlled**
Symptom frequency	≤ 2 days/week, but not > 1 time per day	> 2 days/week or multiple times on ≤ 2 days/week	Throughout the day
Number of nighttime awakenings	≤ 1 time per month	> 1 time per month	> 1 time per week
Frequency of use of SABA to control symptoms	≤ 2 days/week	> 2 days/week	Several times per day
Extent of limitation of normal activity	None	Some	Extreme
Lung Function • Predicted FEV_1 or personal best peak flow • FEV_1/FVC	N/A	N/A	N/A
Exacerbations that require oral systemic corticosteroids Considerations: severity/interval since last exacerbation	0 to 1 time per year	2 to 3 times per year	> 3 times per year
Reduction in lung growth	N/A	N/A	N/A
Treatment-related adverse effects	Side effects vary from none to troublesome; intensity does not correlate to level of control but should be considered		
Recommended Step Therapy Should not replace clinical decision making & individual patient needs	• Maintain current step • Follow up every 1 to 6 months • Consider step-down if well controlled for ≥ 3 months	• Go up 1 step	• Consider short-term course of oral systemic corticosteroid • Step up 1 to 2 steps
Considerations before step-up of therapy	• Factors: adherence, inhaler technique, environmental control • If alternative therapy was used, discontinue & use preferred • Reevaluate every 2 to 6 weeks to get control & every 1 to 6 months to maintain it • If no benefit in 4 to 6 weeks, consider alternative diagnosis or therapy		

Note: SABA = short-acting beta-agonists; FEV_1 = forced expiratory volume in one second; FVC = forced vital capacity.

References: Based on Figure 4-3a, Assessing Asthma Control & Adjusting Therapy in Children 0 to 4 Years of Age; from the National Asthma Education & Prevention Program Expert Panel Report III: Guidelines for the Diagnosis & Management of Asthma. Bethesda, MD: National Heart, Lung, and Blood Institute, 2007. www.nhlbi.nih.gov/guidelines/asthma/asthgdln.htm (Accessed November 2018); Global Strategy for Asthma Management & Prevention, Global Initiative for Asthma (GINA) also may be referenced. http://ginasthma.org/gina-reports/ (Accessed November 2018).

Prepared by Jeanine P. Abrons

Peripheral Brain for the Pharmacist

Adjusting Asthma Therapy in Children Ages 5 to 11

Consideration	Asthma Control and Therapy Adjustment (Based on most impairment, risk, and recall of previous 2 to 4 weeks)		
	Well Controlled	**Not Well Controlled**	**Very Poorly Controlled**
Symptom frequency	≤ 2 days/week, but not > 1 time per day	> 2 days/week or multiple times on ≤ 2 days/week	Throughout the day
Number of nighttime awakenings	≤ 1 time per month	≥ 2 times per month	≥ 2 times per week
Frequency of use of SABA to control symptoms	≤ 2 days/week	> 2 days/week	Several times per day
Extent of limitation of normal activity	None	Some	Extreme
Lung Function • Predicted FEV$_1$ or personal best peak flow • FEV$_1$/FVC	> 80% > 80%	60 to 80% 75 to 80%	< 60% < 75%
Exacerbations that require oral systemic corticosteroids Considerations: severity/interval since last exacerbation	0 to 1 time per year	≥ 2 times per year	≥ 2 times per year
Reduction in lung growth	Requires long-term follow up	Requires long-term follow-up	Requires long-term follow-up
Treatment-related adverse effects	Side effects vary from none to troublesome; intensity not correlate to level of control but should be considered		
Recommended Step Therapy Should not replace clinical decision making & individual patient needs	• Maintain current step • Follow up every 1 to 6 months • Consider step-down if well controlled for ≥ 3 months	• Go up 1 step	• Consider short-term course of oral systemic corticosteroid • Step up 1 to 2 steps
Considerations before step-up of therapy	• Factors: adherence, inhaler technique, environmental control • If alternative therapy was used, discontinue & use preferred • Reevaluate every 2 to 6 weeks to get control & every 1 to 6 months to maintain control • Adjust therapy accordingly		

Note: SABA = short-acting beta-agonists; FEV$_1$ = forced expiratory volume in one second; FVC = forced vital capacity.

References: Based on Figure 4-3b, Classifying Asthma Control & Adjusting Therapy in Children 5 to 11 Years of Age from the National Asthma Education & Prevention Program Expert Panel Report III: Guidelines for the Diagnosis & Management of Asthma. *Bethesda, MD: National Heart, Lung, and Blood Institute, 2007. www.nhlbi.nih.gov/guidelines/asthma/asthgdln.htm (Accessed November 2018);* Global Strategy for Asthma Management & Prevention, Global Initiative for Asthma (GINA) *also may be referenced.* http://ginasthma.org/gina-reports/ (Accessed November 2018).

Prepared by Jeanine P. Abrons

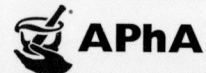

Stepwise Approach for Managing Asthma Long Term in Children Ages 0 to 4

Asthma	Step	Preferred	Alternative	Quick Relief	Notes
Intermittent	1	SABA as needed	N/A	• SABA as needed; intensity depends on symptom severity • Viral respiratory symptoms: SABA q 4 to 6h up to 24h (consider oral corticosteroid if severe) • Frequent use of SABA may mean need to step up	• This process should not replace clinical judgment. • If alternatives don't work, discontinue & use preferred. • Studies in children 0 to 4 years of age are limited.
Persistent	2	Low dose ICS	Cromolyn or montelukast		
	3	Medium dose ICS	N/A		
	4	Medium dose ICS + LABA or montelukast	N/A		
	5	High dose ICS + LABA or montelukast	N/A		
	6	High dose ICS + LABA or montelukast + oral corticosteroids ICS	N/A		

Note: SABA = short-acting beta-agonists; ICS = inhaled corticosteroid; LABA = long-acting beta-agonists; N/A = not applicable.

Stepwise Approach for Managing Asthma Long Term in Children Ages 5 to 11

Asthma	Step	Preferred	Alternative	Quick Relief	Notes
Intermittent	1	SABA as needed	N/A	• SABA as needed; intensity depends on symptom severity • SABA: up to 3 treatments at 20-minute intervals as needed • Frequent use of SABA may mean need to step up	• This process should not replace clinical judgment. • If alternatives don't work, discontinue & use preferred. • Each step: patient education, environmental control, comorbidity management • Steps 2 to 4: consider allergen immunotherapy • Theophylline = less desirable
Persistent	2	Low dose ICS	Cromolyn, LTRA, nedocromil, or theophylline		
	3	Low dose ICS + LABA, LTRA, or theophylline OR medium dose ICS	N/A		
	4	Medium dose ICS + LABA	Medium dose ICS + LTRA or theophylline		
	5	High dose ICS + LABA	High dose ICS + LTRA or theophylline		
	6	High dose ICS + LABA + oral corticosteroids ICS	High dose ICS + LTRA or theophylline + oral cortico-steroid		

Note: SABA = short-acting beta-agonists; ICS = inhaled corticosteroid; LABA = long-acting beta-agonists; LTRA = leukotriene receptor antagonist.

References: Based on Figure 4-1a, Managing Asthma Long Term in Children 0 to 4 Years of Age: Stepwise Approach for Managing Asthma Long Term in Children, 0 to 4 Years of Age; Figure 4-1b, Managing Asthma Long Term in Children 5 to 11 Years of Age: Stepwise Approach for Managing Asthma Long Term in Children 5 to 11 Years of Age from the National Asthma Education & Prevention Program Expert Panel Report III: Guidelines for the Diagnosis & Management of Asthma. Bethesda, MD: National Heart, Lung, and Blood Institute, 2007. www.nhlbi.nih.gov/guidelines/asthma/asthgdln.htm (Accessed November 2018); Global Strategy for Asthma Management & Prevention, Global Initiative for Asthma (GINA) also may be referenced. http://ginasthma.org/gina-reports/ (Accessed November 2018).

Prepared by Jeanine P. Abrons

Initiating Therapy in Youths ≥ 12 Years of Age and Adults with Intermittent Asthma Severity

Consideration	Initiating Therapy with Intermittent Asthma Severity	
	Youth ≥ 12 Years of Age and Adults	
Impairment Normal: FEV_1/FVC. 	**Symptom frequency**	≤ 2 days/week
	Number of nighttime awakenings	≤ 2 times per month
	Frequency of use of SABA to control symptoms	≤ 2 days/week
	Extent of limitation of normal activity	No limitation
	Lung Function • Predicted FEV_1 or personal best peak flow • FEV_1/FVC	• Normal FEV_1 between exacerbations • FEV_1 > 80% predicted • FEV_1/FVC normal
Risk	**Exacerbations that require oral systemic corticosteroids** Considerations: severity & interval since last exacerbation	0 to 1 time per year
Recommendation	**Recommended Step Therapy** Should not replace clinical decision making & individual patient needs	Step 1 Reevaluate in 2 to 6 weeks: level of asthma control

Impairment table:

Age	Normal
8 to 19	85%
20 to 39	80%
40 to 59	75%
60 to 80	70%

Note: SABA = short-acting beta-agonists; FEV_1 = forced expiratory volume in one second; FVC = forced vital capacity.

References: Based on Figure 4-6, Managing Asthma Long Term in Youths ≥ 12 Years of Age from the National Asthma Education & Prevention Program Expert Panel Report III: Guidelines for the Diagnosis & Management of Asthma. Bethesda, MD: National Heart, Lung, and Blood Institute, 2007. www.nhlbi.nih.gov/guidelines/asthma/asthgdln.htm (Accessed November 2018); Global Strategy for Asthma Management & Prevention, Global Initiative for Asthma (GINA) also may be referenced. http://ginasthma.org/gina-reports/ (Accessed November 2018).

Prepared by Jeanine P. Abrons

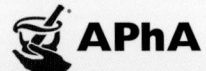

Initiating Therapy in Youths ≥ 12 Years of Age and Adults with Persistent Asthma Severity

Consideration	Initiating Therapy with Persistent Asthma Severity			
	Youth ≥ 12 Years of Age and Adults			
		Mild	Moderate	Severe
Impairment Normal: FEV$_1$/FVC:	Symptom frequency	> 2 days/week, but not daily	Daily	Throughout the day
	Number of nighttime awakenings	3 to 4 times per month	> 1 time per week, but not nightly	Often; 7 times per week
	Frequency of use of SABA to control symptoms	> 2 days/week, but not daily & not > 1 x on any day	Daily	Several times/day
	Extent of limitation of normal activity	Minor limitation	Some limitation	Extreme limitation
	Lung Function • Predicted FEV$_1$ or personal best peak flow • FEV$_1$/FVC	• FEV$_1$ > 80% predicted • FEV$_1$/FVC normal	• FEV$_1$ > 60% but < 80% predicted • FEV$_1$/FVC reduced 5%	• FEV$_1$ < 60% • FEV$_1$/FVC reduced > 5%
Risk	Exacerbations that require oral systemic corticosteroids Considerations: severity/ interval since last exacerbation	≥ 2 times year		
Recommendation	Recommended Step Therapy Should not replace clinical decision making & individual patient needs Reevaluate in 2 to 6 weeks: level of asthma control	Step 2	Step 3	Steps 4 or 5
			Consider short course of oral systemic corticosteroids	

Impairment Normal: FEV$_1$/FVC age table:

Age	Normal
8 to 19	85%
20 to 39	80%
40 to 59	75%
60 to 80	70%

Note: SABA = short-acting beta-agonists; FEV$_1$ = forced expiratory volume in one second; FVC = forced vital capacity.

References: Based on Figure 4-6, Managing Asthma Long Term in Youths ≥12 Years of Age from the National Asthma Education & Prevention Program Expert Panel Report III: Guidelines for the Diagnosis & Management of Asthma. Bethesda, MD: National Heart, Lung, and Blood Institute, 2007. www.nhlbi.nih.gov/guidelines/asthma/asthgdln.htm (Accessed November 2018); Global Strategy for Asthma Management & Prevention, Global Initiative for Asthma (GINA) also may be referenced. http://ginasthma.org/gina-reports/ (Accessed November 2018).

Prepared by Jeanine P. Abrons

Assessing Therapy in Youths ≥ 12 Years of Age and Adults Based on Asthma Control

Level of Control	Symptom Frequency	Awake at Night	Activity Limits	Symptom Control (SABA Use)	FEV₁/Peak Flow (Predicted)*	Corticosteroid Use	Treatment
Well controlled	≤ 2 days/week	≤ 2 times per month	None	≤ 2 days/week	> 80%	0 to 1 time per year	• Keep up current step & control • Follow up 1 to 6 months • Step down if control for 3 months
Not controlled	> 2 days/week	1 to 3 times per week	Some	> 2 days/week	60 to 80%	≥ 2 times per year	• 1 step up • Follow-up in 2 to 6 weeks • Consider other options if side effects
Very poorly controlled	Throughout day	≥ 4 times per week	Extreme	Several times daily	< 60%	≥ 2 times per year	• May use short course of oral steroid • 1 to 2 steps up • Follow up in 2 weeks • Consider other options if side effects

*Note: SABA = short-acting beta-agonists; FEV₁ = forced expiratory volume in one second; * = or personal best*

Stepwise Approach for Managing Asthma Long Term in Youths ≥ 12 Years of Age and Adults

Asthma	Step	Preferred	Alternative or Addition	Quick Relief	Notes
Intermittent	1	SABA as needed	N/A	• SABA as needed: intensity depends on symptom severity • SABA: up to 3 treatments at 20-minute intervals as needed • Frequent use of SABA may mean need to step up	• This process should not replace clinical judgment. • If alternatives don't work, discontinue & use preferred. • Each step: patient education, environmental control, comorbidity management • Steps 2 to 4: consider allergen immunotherapy • Theophylline = less desirable
Persistent	2	Low dose ICS	**Alternative:** cromolyn, LTRA, nedocromil, or theophylline		
	3	Low dose ICS + LABA OR medium dose ICS	**Alternative:** low dose ICS + LABA, LTRA, theophylline, or zileuton		
	4	Medium dose ICS + LABA	**Alternative:** medium dose ICS + LTRA, theophylline, or zileuton		
	5	High dose ICS + LABA	**Addition:** consider omalizumab in patients with allergies		
	6	High dose ICS + LABA + oral corticosteroids	**Addition:** consider omalizumab in patients with allergies		

Note: SABA = short-acting beta-agonists; ICS = inhaled corticosteroid; LABA = long-acting beta-agonist; LTRA = leukotriene receptor antagonist; N/A = not applicable.

References: Based on Figure 4-7, Assessing and Adjusting Therapy in Youths ≥ 12 Years of Age and Adults and on Figure 4-5, Stepwise Approach for Managing Asthma Long Term in Youths ≥ 12 Years of Age and Adults from the National Asthma Education & Prevention Program Expert Panel Report III: Guidelines for the Diagnosis & Management of Asthma. Bethesda, MD: National Heart, Lung, and Blood Institute, 2007. www.nhlbi.nih.gov/guidelines/asthma/asthgdln.htm [Accessed November 2018]; Global Strategy for Asthma Management & Prevention, Global Initiative for Asthma (GINA) also may be referenced: http://ginasthma.org/gina-reports/ [Accessed November 2018].

Prepared by Jeanine P. Abrons

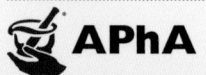

Assessment of Airflow Limitation/Symptoms in Chronic Obstructive Pulmonary Disease (COPD)

COPD Airflow Limitation

GOLD Class	Degree of Limitation	FEV_1
1	Mild	$FEV_1 \geq 80\%$ predicted
2	Moderate	$50\% \leq FEV_1 < 80\%$ predicted
3	Severe	$30\% \leq FEV_1 < 50\%$ predicted
4	Very severe	$FEV_1 < 30\%$ predicted

Symptom (Dyspnea)

mMRC Grade	Description of Limitation
0	Only gets breathless with strenuous activity
1	Gets short of breath when hurrying on level ground or walking slightly uphill
2	Walks slower than others of age on level ground due to breathlessness or has to stop for breath when walking at own pace on level ground
3	Stops for breath when walking ~ 100 meters or after few minutes walking on level ground
4	Too breathless to leave house or when dressing or undressing

CAT Element	Description of Limitation
Cough	Never (0) to All the time (5)
Phlegm (Mucus)	None in chest (0) to Completely full of phlegm (5)
Chest tightness	Not tight at all (0) to Very tight (5)
Hill or 1 flight of stairs	Not breathless while walking (0) to Very breathless while walking (5)
Limits activity at home	Not limited (0) to Very limited (5)
Confidence leaving home	Confident (0) to Not confident (5)
Sleeping	Sleep soundly (0) to Don't sleep soundly (5)
Energy	Have lots (0) to No energy (5) at all

Notes: FEV = forced expiratory volume; correlation between FEV_1, symptoms, & health status impairment is weak. Formal symptom assessment also required. Spirometric cut-points are for simplicity; To ↓ variability, perform spirometry after ≥ 1 dose of short-acting inhaled bronchodilator; mMRC = modified British Medical Research Council; CAT = COPD Assessment Test; Notes: Post-bronchodilator FEV₁/FVC < 0.70 confirms airflow limitation.

References: CAT = Jones et al. ERJ 2009;34(3);648-54; mMRC = Fletcher CM. BMJ 1960;2018 GOLD Guidelines available at https://goldcopd.org/wp-content/uploads/2017/11/GOLD-2018-v6.0-FINAL-revised-20-Nov_WMS.pdf (Accessed November 2018)

Use these assessments to determine ABCD Groups in COPD.

Reference: From the Global Strategy for Diagnosis, Management and Prevention of COPD 2018 ©.

Prepared by Jeanine P Abrons and Anh Luong

Assessment to Determine ABCD Groups in Chronic Obstructive Pulmonary Disease (COPD)

STEP 1: Confirm Diagnosis	STEP 2: Assess Airflow Limitation/ Symptom Severity			STEP 3: Record Exacerbation History			STEP 4: Combine Symptom Assessment/ Exacerbation Risk	
• Use spirometry to define spirometric grade (airflow limits) • Postbronchodilator FEV_1/FVC < 0.70 confirms airflow limitation	• Classify airflow limitation severity (use GOLD 1 to 4) • Assess symptoms (use mMRC Scale & CAT Assessment)			• Prior exacerbation prevalence/severity • Number of prior hospitalizations/ exacerbation risk			Assessment of symptoms/risk of exacerbation	
With Presence of Key Indicators	Class	Description		Class	Description		GOLD Group	Description
• Dyspnea (progressive; worse with exercise; persistent) • Chronic cough (intermittent; unproductive; recurrent wheeze) • Chronic sputum • Recurrent lower respiratory tract infections • History of risk factors (host factors, tobacco smoke, smoke, occupational exposures) • Family history and/or childhood factors (low birthweight, childhood respiratory infections)	**Low Severity**	• mMRC ≤ 1 OR • CAT ≤ 9		**Lower Risk**	0 or 1 exacerbation (not leading to hospital admission in last 12 months)		A	• Low symptom severity • Low exacerbation risk
							B	• High symptom severity • Low exacerbation risk
	High Severity	• mMRC ≥ 2 OR • CAT ≥ 10		**Higher Risk**	≥ 2 exacerbations or any resulting in hospital admission in past 12 months		C	• Low symptom severity • High exacerbation risk
							D	• High symptom severity • High exacerbation risk

Reference: 2018 GOLD Guidelines available at: https://goldcopd.org/wp-content/uploads/2017/11/GOLD-2018-v6.0-FINAL-revised-20-Nov_WMS.pdf (Accessed November 2018).

Prepared by Jeanine P. Abrons and Anh Luong

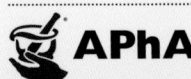

Community-Acquired Pneumonia (CAP) Management

Causative Bacteria		Respiratory Viruses	
Streptococcus pneumoniae	Chlamydophila pneumonia	Influenza A & B	Rhinoviruses
Haemophilus influenza	Legionella species	Parainfluenza viruses	Adenoviruses
Moraxella catarrhalis	Mycoplasma pneumonia	Respiratory syncytial virus	Human bocaviruses
Other gram (-) bacilli	Staphylococcus aurea		

Signs and Symptoms		Predisposing Risk Factors	
Pulmonary signs & symptoms (Cough [with or without sputum production]); dyspnea; pleuritic chest pain; tachypnea; ↑ effort in breathing; crackles or rales; hypoxemia; sputum production)		Age > 65	Immunosuppressive conditions
		Smoking	Alcoholism
		Viral respiratory tract infections	Chronic Obstructive Pulmonary Disease (COPD)
Systemic signs & symptoms (Fever; chills; fatigue; malaise; tachycardia; rise in inflammatory markers (e.g., ESR; CRP)**		Chronic comorbidities (Chronic cardiovascular, or cerebrovascular disease, diabetes, and dementia);	Lung function changes (e.g., Cystic fibrosis; Karagener syndrome; Young syndrome; immotile cilia syndrome; Bioterrorism [anthrax; tularemia; plague])
Radiographic findings on Chest X-ray (Opacities; lobar consolidations; interstitial infiltrates)			

How Is CAP Diagnosed?	How Is the Severity of CAP Evaluated?
• Presence of clinically compatible signs/symptoms with radiographic findings • Blood cultures (x2) and/or expectorated sputum samples for culture and gram stain* • Legionella urinary antigen assays and cultures: Obtain serum procalcitonin level if culture results are negative	Can be made through either CURB-65 (See notes for criteria) or Pneumonia Severity Index (PSI; also known as the PORT score)

*Note: Always consider institution-specific susceptibilities; *C = confusion; U = urea > 20 mg/dL; R = respiratory rate ≥ 30 breaths/minute; B = blood pressure (low systolic < 90 or diastolic ≤ 60 mmHg); A = age ≥ 65) – Score of 3 or > predicts higher mortality. **Erythrocyte sedimentation rate; CRP = C-reactive protein*

Treatment of Community-Acquired Pneumonia (CAP)

Setting/Situation	Treatment (Drug/Duration)
Level 1): Ambulatory Care (Empiric Options)—PSI scores of I to II and CURB-65 scores of 0 (or CURB-65 score of 1 if age >65)	
Previously healthy and no risk factors for drug-resistant *S. pneumoniae* (DRSP) infection	• Doxycycline for 7 to 10 days
	• Macrolide (clarithromycin; azithromycin; erythromycin) for 7 to 10 days
With comorbidity (chronic heart, lung, or liver disease; diabetes; alcoholism; immunosuppression; malignancies, asplenia, or other risks for drug resistant *S. pneumoniae* infection) or recent antibiotic therapy (within past 3 months)	• Fluoroquinolone (moxifloxacin, gemifloxacin, or levofloxacin 750mg)
	• β-lactam & Macrolide: high-dose amoxicillin (1 g three times daily) or amoxicillin clavulanate (2 g two times daily) preferred; alternatives = ceftriaxone; cefuroxime, & doxycycline
Hospitalized Patient (Empiric/Nonintensive Care Unit)—Patients SpO2 < 92% on room air with significant change from baseline OR with PSI scores of ≥ III & CURB-65 scores ≥ 1 (or CURB-65 score ≥ 2 if age >65)	
Therapy expanded to include *S. aureus* and gram (-) bacilli in addition to typical pathogens	• Respiratory fluoroquinolone (monotherapy) for 7 to 10 days
	• β-lactam (e.g., ceftriaxone, cefotaxime, or cefpodoxime (500 mg 2 times daily)) & macrolide (alternative = doxycycline) for 7 to 10 days
	• β-lactam + either azithromycin or fluoroquinolone
	• Alternative management for pseudomonas
Patients without Methicillin-Resistant *S. Aureus* (MRSA) or risk factors for pseudomonas	• Combo therapy with a β-lactam plus either macrolide or doxycycline OR
	• Monotherapy with respiratory fluoroquinolone
Patients with risk factors for pseudomonas	• Antipseudomonal β-lactam (e.g., piperacillin-tazobactam, cefepime, ceftazidime, meropenem, or imipenem) + antipseudomonal fluoroquinolone (e.g., ciprofloxacin or levofloxacin 750 mg) OR
	• β-lactam + aminoglycoside & azithromycin OR
	• β-lactam + aminoglycoside & fluoroquinolone
Patients with risk factors for MRSA	• Add an agent with anti-MRSA activity: vancomycin (trough = 15 to 20 ug/mL or 15 mg/kg) or linezolid
Pathogen Specific Treatment Options	
S. pneumoniae	• Amoxicillin; ceftriaxone; cefotaxime; macrolide; fluoroquinolone
MSSA	• Oxacillin; nafcillin
Mycoplasma or chlamydia	• Macrolide or doxycycline for 7 days
H. influenzae	• Doxycycline; 2nd or 3rd generation cephalosporin or fluroquinolone x 1 to 2 weeks

Notes: Patients with CAP should be treated for a min of 5 days, should be afebrile for 48–72 h, and should have no > 1 CAP-associated sign of clinical instability; MSSA = Methicillin-sensitive S. Aureues. Additional management strategies for ICU patients not listed on this card.

Sample references: Alterations in therapeutic selection made with severe beta lactam allergy. Jain S, Self WH, Wunderink RG, et al. Community-Acquired Pneumonia Requiring Hospitalization among U.S. Adults. N Engl J Med 2015; 373:415; Mandell LA, Wunderink RG, Anzueto A, et al. Infectious Diseases Society of America/American Thoracic Society consensus guidelines on the management of community-acquired pneumonia in adults. Clin Infect Dis 2007; 44 Suppl 2:S27.

Hospital-Acquired Pneumonia (HAP) Management

Common Pathogens

❏ **S. aureus**
  ❏ Methicillin-resistant *S. Aureus* (MRSA)
  ❏ Methicillin-sensitive *S. Aureus* (MSSA)

❏ **Gram-negative bacilli**
  ❏ *Klebsiella*
  ❏ *Pseudomonas aeruginosa*
  ❏ *Enterobacter*
  ❏ *S. maltophilia*
  ❏ *E. coli*
  ❏ *Acinetobacter* spp.

❏ *Legionella* spp.

❏ **Viruses**
  ❏ Influenza
  ❏ RSV
  ❏ Parainfluenza

❏ **Anaerobes**

Notes: Most common are MRSA and gram-negative bacilli. Most difficult to treat are P. aeruginosa & Acinetobacter.

Empiric Treatment

Based on patient's risk of multidrug resistance (MDR):
❏ Receipt of intravenous antibiotics during prior 90 days
❏ High risk of mortality

Additional risk factors for Pseudomonas

❏ Hospitalization in unit where >10% of gram-negative isolates are resistant to an agent being considered for monotherapy
❏ Patient in septic shock
❏ Patient with structural lung disease (bronchiectasis; cystic fibrosis)

Additional risk factors for MRSA

❏ Hospitalization in unit where >20% of *S. aureus* isolates are methicillin resistant
❏ Prevalence of MRSA unknown

Note: Refer to your institution's local susceptibilities for further guidance on empiric treatment.

Reference: Chart based on Tables 4 and 5 of ATS/IDSA Guidelines

Empiric Therapy

NOT AT HIGH RISK of Mortality and NO FACTORS Increasing Likelihood of Multidrug Resistant (MDR) Pathogens (CHOOSE ONE)

Medication	Dose[a]
Piperacillin/tazobactam[b]	4.5 g IV q6h
Cefepime	2 g IV q8h
Levofloxacin	750 mg IV daily
Imipenem[b]	500 mg IV q6h
Meropenem[b]	1 g IV q8h

CHOOSE TWO for MDR and/or Pseudomonas Risk (CHOOSE ONE β-lactam/Carbapenem and ONE from Another Class)

Medication	Dose[a]
Piperacillin/tazobactam[b]	4.5 g IV q6h
Cefepime	2 g IV q8h
Ceftazidime	2 g IV q8h
Levofloxacin	750 mg IV daily
Ciprofloxacin	400 mg IV q8h
Imipenem[b]	500 mg IV q6h
Meropenem[b]	1g IV q8h
Amikacin	15 to 20 mg/kg IV daily
Gentamicin	5 to 7 mg/kg IV daily
Tobramycin	5 to 7 mg/kg IV daily
Aztreonam	2 g IV q8h

Add for MDR and/or MRSA Risk (CHOOSE ONE)

Vancomycin[c]	15 mg/kg IV q8 to 12h Achieve trough of 15 to 20 mg/mL (consider loading dose of 25 to 30 mg/kg IV x 1 for severe illness)
Linezolid	600 mg IV q12h

a. Alternate dosing regimens using pharmacokinetic/pharmacodynamic (PK/PD) data may be used.
b. Extended infusions may be appropriate.
c. Area under the curve (AUC) targets of 400–600 mg hr/L may be used instead of trough goals

Reference: Chart based on Table 4 of 2016 IDSA HAP/VAP Guidelines.

Hospital-Acquired Pneumonia (HAP) Management *(continued)*

Risk Reduction

- Effective infection control measures (education; compliance; isolation)
- Surveillance of infections to identify, quantify, and prepare
- Intubation/mechanical ventilation avoidance and duration reduction when possible (guidance exists on preferred type of intubation and tubes)
- Patient positioning (semirecumbent positioning)
- Modulation of oropharyngeal colonization by combinations of antibiotics (oral) with or without systemic therapy or selective decontamination of digestive tract (SDD)
- Consideration of risk associated with stress ulcer prophylaxis regimen or chronic proton pump inhibitor therapy
- Consideration of type of transfusion (undetermined)
- Blood glucose management

References

- Institution Specific Formulary http://www.hopkinsguides.com/hopkins/ub
- Kalil AC, Metersky ML, Klompas M, Muscedere J, Sweeney DA, et al. Management of Adults with Hospital-acquired and Ventilator-associated Pneumonia: 2016 Clinical Practice Guidelines by the Infectious Diseases Society of America and the American Thoracic Society. *Clinical Infectious Diseases* 2016; 63(5):e61-111. cid.oxfordjournals.org/content/early/2016/07/06/cid.ciw353.

Prepared by Jeanine P. Abrons, Ben Lomaestro, and Bryan P. White
Additional card updates with Adrienne Rouiller and Bryan P. White

---

HAP or VAP Suspected

Obtain lower respiratory tract (LRT) sample for culture and microscopy

↓

Unless there is both a low clinical suspicion for pneumonia and negative microscopy of LRT sample, begin empiric antimicrobial therapy using guideline algorithm and local microbiologic data.

Days 2 and 3:
Check cultures: assess clinical response (e.g., temperature, white blood cell, chest x-ray, purulent sputum).

↓

Clinical improvement in 48 to 72 hours

NO

Culture –	Culture +
Search for other pathogens, complications, diagnoses, or sites of infection	Adjust antibiotic therapy; search for other pathogens, complications, diagnoses, or other sites of infection

YES

Culture –	Culture +
Consider stopping antibiotics	De-escalate antibiotics (when possible). Consider treating for 7 to 8 days; then reassess.

Suggested treatment duration of 7 days

Reference: Based on Figure 1 of ATS/IDSA Guidelines

Note: VAP = ventilator-associated pneumonia.

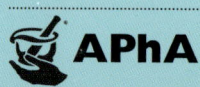

APhA

Aminoglycosides: Traditional Considerations and Dosing in Adults

General Information

- Fight bacteria by interrupting bacterial protein synthesis.
- Bactericidal against gram-negative aerobic organisms including *Pseudomonas*
- Active against *Staphylococci* but inactive against *Streptococci*
- Synergistic with some penicillins (including ampicillin) and vancomycin against *Enterococci*
- Demonstrate concentration-dependent killing
- Have a significant postantibiotic effect
- Amount in the tissue accumulates over time contributing to toxicity
- Average volume of distribution in otherwise healthy adults = 0.26 L/kg (range 0.2 to 0.3)
- Does not distribute to adipose tissue; obese patients require a correction in weight used for V_d (patients with cystic fibrosis; and ascites also may require corrections)
- Important adverse effects: nephrotoxicity; ototoxicity; neuromuscular blockage; rash
- Elimination closely correlated with creatinine clearance

Aminoglycoside Area	Notes/Discussion
Target Therapeutic Levels (Peaks)	• Gentamicin/tobramycin: 4 to 8 mcg/mL (normal); urinary tract infection: 4 to 5 mcg/mL; endocarditis: 3 to 4 mcg/mL; cystic fibrosis: 8 to 10 mcg/mL • Amikacin: 20 to 25 mcg/mL (traditional dosing); 40 to 100 mcg/mL (single daily dose)
Initial or Maintenance Dose	• Doses of aminoglycosides must be individualized based on the patient characteristics such as age, weight, renal function, and infection treated. • See side 2 of card for single daily dosing strategy; single daily dosing shown to have lower incidence & longer time to onset of nephrotoxicity than traditional dosing. • Gentamicin traditional dosing of adults (not single daily dosing) is 3 to 5 mg/kg IV or IM divided every 8 hours until over the age of 60 (then, 3 mg/kg divided every 12 hours) • Tobramycin traditional dosing of adults: 1 to 2 mg/kg IV over 30 minutes every 8 hours • Amikacin traditional dosing of adults: 5 mg/kg IV over 30 min every 8 hours or 7.5 mg/kg over 30 min every 12 hours • Dose adjustments must be made based on renal function. • Other certain populations also require dosage adjustments (e.g., based on postmenstrual age (gentamicin), for cystic fibrosis, for hemodialysis (postdialysis dosing) • This dosing reflects adult dosing and not dosing used on neonatal or pediatric patient population.
Other Monitoring (Beyond peak and trough levels)	<table><tr><td>**Monitoring Parameter**</td></tr><tr><td>Blood urea nitrogen (BUN)</td></tr><tr><td>Serum creatinine</td></tr><tr><td>Weight</td></tr><tr><td>Hearing</td></tr></table>
Recommendations for Monitoring Levels	• Ensure proper timing of sampling to enable accurate interpretation of levels. Note time samples were drawn and when infusions were started and stopped. • Sampling for peak in traditional dosing completed 20 to 30 minutes following infusion; 1 hour for single daily dosing.

Prepared by Ben Lomaestro and Bryan P. White

Commonly Used Abbreviations

Term	Definition	Term	Definition
TBW	total body weight	CrCl	creatinine clearance in mL/min
IBW	ideal body weight	SCr	serum creatinine
NS	normal saline		

Aminoglycosides: Single Daily Dosing

Step	Description
1) Initial Aminoglycoside Dose Given as a Single Daily Dose (SDD):	Suggested initial dosing

Drug	DOSE	
	Normal	**Critically Ill/Septic Patient**
Gentamicin	6 mg/kg	7 mg/kg
Tobramycin	6 mg/kg	7 mg/kg
Amikacin	24 mg/kg	30 to 40 mg/kg

Use TBW unless patient weight is > 40% above the IBW; then consider use of adjusted body weight or ideal body weight.

Step	Description
2) Determination of Dosing Interval	• Dosing interval is based upon estimated CrCl.

$$CrCl = \frac{(140 - age) \times IBW \text{ (in kg)} \times (0.85 \text{ in females})}{(72 \times SCr)}$$

• Determine the initial dosing interval

Calculated CrCl	Initial Dosing Interval
60 mL/min or >	Every 24 hours
40–60 mL/min	X1 dose based on drug levels

Step	Description
3) Administration	• Administration time over 1 hour or consult institution specific guidelines. • Following infusion with a flush of 50 mL NS to ensure dose administered. • Record actual start and stop time.
4) Serum Concentration Monitoring	• Obtain PEAK concentration 1 hour after END of infusion. • Obtain a second or RANDOM concentration between 8 and 10 hours after END of infusion. • Record ACTUAL time sampled. • Record ACTUAL start and stop time of infusion and state "single dose interval." • Trough levels should be undetectable with SDD.
5) Dosage/ Regimen Adjustment Based on Table	• Adjust dosage regimen based on serum concentrations. Dosage changes result in proportional changes in serum concentrations. PEAK (1 hour post infusion) concentration interpretation (use higher level for resistant organisms)

Drug	Recommended Action Based on PEAK Concentration	
Gentamicin and Tobramycin	Concentration	Course of Action
	7 mg/kg levels also can be evaluated based on the Hartford nomogram	
	> 25 mcg/mL	Reduce dose to achieve peak < 25 mcg/mL
	10 to 25 mcg/mL	Maintain dose
	< 10 mcg/mL	Increase dose to achieve level > 10 mcg/mL
Amikacin	Concentration	Course of Action
	> 100 mcg/mL	Reduce dose to achieve first level < 100 mcg/mL
	40 to 100 mcg/mL	Maintain dose
	< 40 mcg/mL	Increase dose to achieve level > 40 mcg/mL

Reference: Nicolau DP, Freeman CD, Belliveau PP, Nightingale CH, Ross JW, Quintiliani R. Experience with a once-daily aminoglycoside program administered to 2,184 adult patients. Antimicrob Agents Chemother. 1995;39(3):650-5.

Note: Use institution-specific dosing guidelines if available. For sbbreviations, see previous page.

Prepared by Ben Lomaestro and Bryan P. White; updated by Bryan P. White

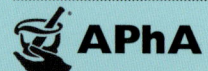

Vancomycin: Considerations and Dosing in Adults

Dosing Consideration	Notes/Discussion
Target Therapeutic Troughs	• Other indications: 10 to 15 mcg/mL • Bacteremia, meningitis, osteomyelitis, pneumonia, endocarditis, and necrotizing fasciitis: 15 to 20 mcg/mL
Initial or Maintenance Dose (For *C.difficile* colitis dosing—See side 2 of card) *= Administer longer than 1 hour for doses > 1 g*	• Typical dosing is based upon actual body weight. • **In morbidly obese adults:** Use "adjusted body weight" = *IBW + 0.4 times the difference between actual body weight and IBW (morbid obesity may be defined by kg or BMI > 40)*

Population	Dosing
Individuals < 65 Years of Age	• **Trough Targets of 10 to 15 mcg/mL:** 15 mg/kg or 1 g intravenous (IV) every 8 to 12 hours over at least 1 hour*. Frequency based on renal function (see below). • **Trough Concentrations of 15 to 20 mcg/mL:** For serious infections, consider loading with 20 to 30 mg/kg (may consider max 3 g/dose) IV at rate of 1 g/hour x 1. Then, 15 to 20 mg/kg IV (max 2 g/dose) at a rate 1 g/hour every 8 to 12 hours.
Individuals > 65 Years of Age	• **Trough Targets of 10 to 15 mcg/mL:** 15 mg/kg or 1 g IV over at least 1 hour* No more often than every 12 hours initially—if CrCl < 50 mL/min give every 24 hours; If CrCl < 20 mL/min, give initial dose and base subsequent doses on drug levels. • **Trough Concentrations of 15 to 20 mcg/mL:** Consider loading with 20 to 30 mg/kg IV at a rate of 1 g/hour* then 15 to 20 mg/kg at 1 g/hour or slower at frequency adjusted for renal function (see below).

Dose Adjustments Made Based on Renal Impairment		
> 100	Every 8 to 12 hours (If > 65 years start with every 12 hour dosing)	**10 to 19**	Every 24 to 48 hours (monitor levels)
80 to 99	Every 8 to 12 hours (If > 65 years start with every 12 hour dosing)	**Below 10**	750 mg to 1 g ONCE (monitor levels)
50 to 79	Every 12 hours	**Hemodialysis**	Based on levels and targeting trough - see reference for more information
30 to 49	Every 24 hours	**CRRT**	Single initial dose based on target and weight as above with monitoring of random levels
20 to 29	Every 24 hours		

Adverse Effects	• Rapid infusions may produce flushing or rash (red man syndrome) possibly accompanied by hypotension due to release of histamine. Slow infusions over 1 hour to reduce risk. Local reactions at site of administration; nephrotoxicity; ototoxicity; leukopenia; eosinophilia; thrombocytopenia; chills; nausea; fever muscle aches; autoimmune reactions

Notes on Use and Interpretation:
• Always refer to local institutional practices/recommendations of antimicrobial stewardship when available.
• For larger infusions, administer no faster than 1 g/hour to reduce risk of red man syndrome.
• Variations in dosing may exist dependent on institution. For example, use of 2 g max loading dose.

Prepared by Ben Lomaestro and Bryan P. White

Sampling Time

Trough: 1 hour or less before next dose; generally draw 1st trough prior to 3rd or 4th dose; trough monitoring may not accurately reflect optimal area under the curve (AUC) exposure.

References

Crew P, Heintz SJ, Heintz BH. Vancomycin dosing and monitoring for patients with end-stage renal disease receiving intermittent hemodialysis. *Am J Health Syst Pharm.* 2015;72(21):1856-64.

Vancomycin: General Information and Dosing (PO/IV) for *C. difficile* Colitis

General Information:

Vancomycin

- Glycopeptide antimicrobial effective against gram-positive organisms including *Streptococci, Staphylococci* (including methicillin-resistant *Staphylococcus aureus* [MRSA]) and coagulase-negative *Staphylococci*.
- Bacteriostatic against *Enterococci*; bactericidal against *Corynebacterium* and *Clostridia*.
- Use by mouth or per rectum for *C. difficile* colitis.
- Pregnancy Category: C
- Lactation: considered safe
- Critical drug interactions: Use caution in combining IV vancomycin with nephrotoxic or ototoxic agents such as aminoglycosides piperacillin/tazobactam, amphotericin B and cisplatin; cholestyramine and colestipol bind to vancomycin and are contraindicated when using vancomycin for *C. difficile* colitis.

C. difficile Colitis Category	Corresponding Vancomycin Dosing (From IDSA Guidelines)
Initial Episode, Mild to Severe	• Vancomycin 125 mg by mouth every 6 hours for 10 days. • Metronidazole 500 mg every 8 hours for 10 days may be used if oral vancomycin and fidaxomicin are not available.
Initial Episode, Fulminant/ICU	• 500 mg every 6 hours (4 times per day) by mouth or nasogastric tube plus metronidazole 500 mg every 8 hours IV. If complete ileum, consider adding rectal installation of vancomycin.
Initial/First Recurrence	• Use vancomycin taper regimen: 125 mg 4 times per day for 10–14 days 2 times per week for 1 week, 1 time per day for 1 week, and then every 2 or 4 days for 2–8 weeks.
Severe/Complicated or ICU	• 500 mg by mouth every 6 hours plus metronidazole 500 mg IV every 8 hours and if patient has ileus rectal vancomycin
Recurrent (Second and Greater)	• Fidaxomicin 200 mg PO twice daily for 10 days should be considered for 2nd recurrence if a patient has failed vancomycin and vancomycin taper. Fecal microbiota transplantation should be considered for the 3rd recurrence.
Clinical Definition	**Supportive Clinical Data from *C. difficile* Guidelines**
Initial episode; mild to moderate	• Leukocytosis with white blood cells (WBC) of 15,000 cells/μL or **lower** and SCr level <1.5 times premorbid level
Initial episode; severe	• Leukocytosis with WBCs of 15,000 cells/μL or higher and SCr ≥ 1.5 times premorbid level
Initial episode; severe complicated	• Hypotension or shock, ileus, or megacolon

Recommended Resources/References

- *C. difficile* guidelines available at: Infectious Disease Society of America (IDSA): http://www.idsociety.org.
- Kullar R, Leonard SN, Davis SL, Delgado G, Pogue JM et al. Validation of the effectiveness of vancomycin nomogram in achieving target trough concentrations of 15 to 20 mg/L Suggested by the Vancomycin Consensus Guidelines. *Pharmacotherapy*, 2011. 31(5): 441–48.
- Surawicz CM, Brandt LJ, Binion DG et al. Guidelines for diagnosis, treatment, and prevention of Clostridium difficile infections. *Am J Gastroenterol* 2013;108:478-98.

Prepared by Ben Lomaestro and Bryan P. White

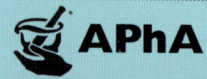
APhA

Gram Stain Interpretation – GRAM + RESULT

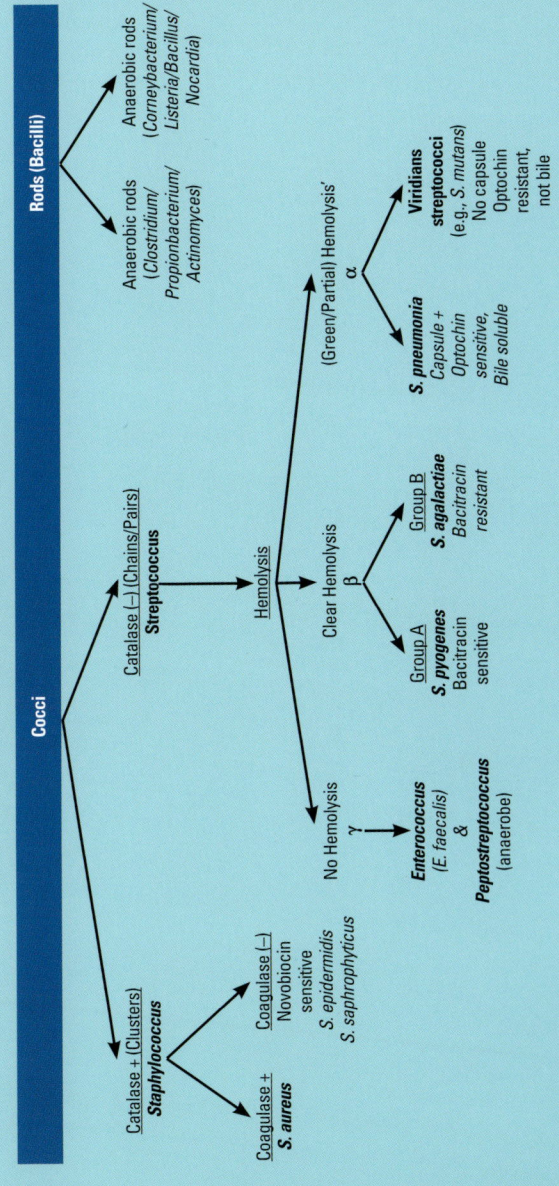

Cocci

Catalase + (Clusters)
Staphylococcus

- **Coagulase +**
  S. aureus
- **Coagulase (–)**
  Novobiocin
  sensitive
  S. epidermidis
  S. saphrophyticus

Catalase (–) (Chains/Pairs)
Streptococcus

Hemolysis

- **No Hemolysis**
  γ
  Enterococcus
  (*E. faecalis*)
  &
  Peptostreptococcus
  (anaerobe)
- **Clear Hemolysis**
  β
  - Group A
    S. pyogenes
    Bacitracin
    sensitive
  - Group B
    S. agalactiae
    Bacitracin
    resistant
- **(Green/Partial) Hemolysis'**
  α
  - ***S. pneumonia***
    Capsule +
    Optochin
    sensitive,
    Bile soluble
  - ***Viridians***
    streptococci
    (e.g., *S. mutans*)
    No capsule
    Optochin
    resistant,
    not bile

Rods (Bacilli)

- Anaerobic rods
  (*Clostridium/*
  Propionbacterium/
  Actinomyces)
- Anaerobic rods
  (*Corneybacterium/*
  Listeria/Bacillus/
  Nocardia)

Modified Based on:
Gomella LG, Haist ST. Clinician's Pocket Reference, 11th Edition; Nebraska Medicine Antimicrobial & Clinical Microbiology Guidebook. Available at: https://www.nebraskamed.com/sites/default/files/documents/for-providers/asp/ID_guidebook_updated-5-2012.pdf. Accessed 14 November 2018.

Gram Stain Interpretation – GRAM – RESULT

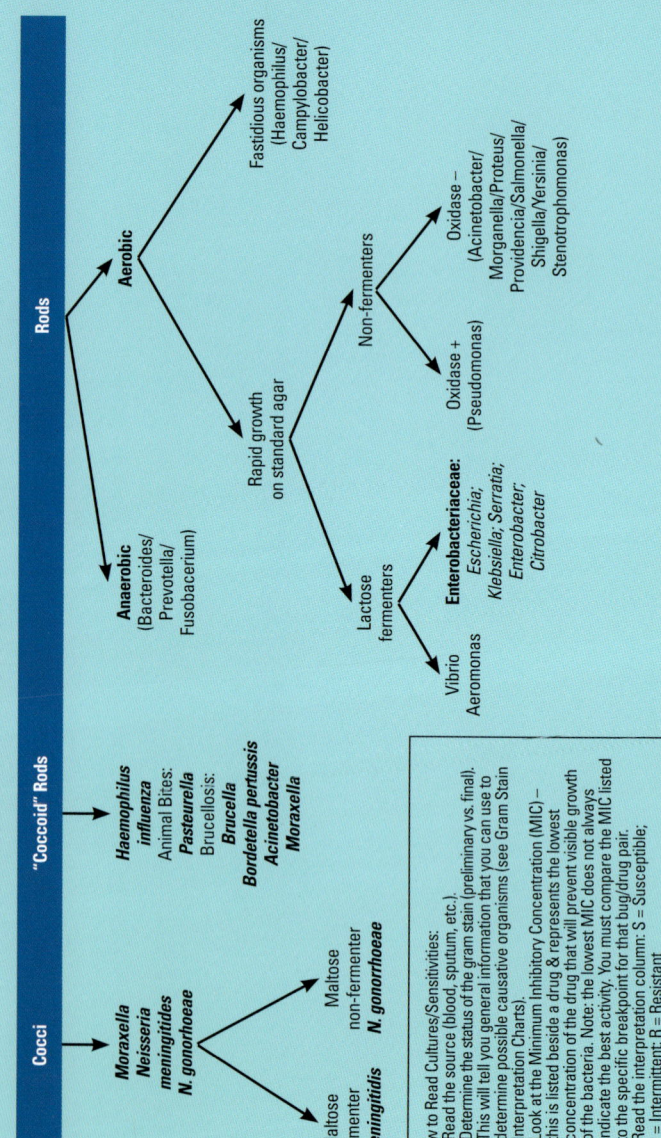

Cocci

Moraxella
Neisseria
meningitides
N. gonorrhoeae

Maltose fermenter
N. meningitidis

Maltose non-fermenter
N. gonorrhoeae

"Coccoid" Rods

Haemophilus
influenza
Animal Bites:
Pasteurella
Brucellosis:
Brucella
Bordetella pertussis
Acinetobacter
Moraxella

Rods

Aerobic

Fastidious organisms
(Haemophilus/
Campylobacter/
Helicobacter)

Rapid growth
on standard agar

Non-fermenters

Oxidase –
(Acinetobacter/
Morganella/Proteus/
Providencia/Salmonella/
Shigella/Yersinia/
Stenotrophomonas)

Oxidase +
(Pseudomonas)

Lactose
fermenters

Enterobacteriaceae:
Escherichia;
Klebsiella; Serratia;
Enterobacter;
Citrobacter

Vibrio
Aeromonas

Anaerobic
(Bacteroides/
Prevotella/
Fusobacerium)

How to Read Cultures/Sensitivities:
1) Read the source (blood, sputum, etc.).
2) Determine the status of the gram stain (preliminary vs. final).
   This will tell you general information that you can use to
   determine possible causative organisms (see Gram Stain
   Interpretation Charts).
3) Look at the Minimum Inhibitory Concentration (MIC) –
   this is listed beside a drug & represents the lowest
   concentration of the drug that will prevent visible growth
   of the bacteria. Note: the lowest MIC does not always
   indicate the best activity. You must compare the MIC listed
   to the specific breakpoint for that bug/drug pair.
4) Read the interpretation column: S = Susceptible;
   I = Intermittent; R = Resistant

Modified Based on:
Gomella LG, Haist ST: Clinician's Pocket Reference, 11th Edition & Guzman OE. Chapter 32 – Antibiotic Streamlining. Competence Assessment Tools for Health-System Pharmacies. Available at:
https://www.ashp.org/-/media/store-files/p4023-sample-chapter-32.ashx. Nebraska Medicine Antimicrobial Guide: https://www.nebraskamed.com/sites/default/files/documents/for-providers/
asp/ID_guidebook_updated-5-2012.pdf (Accessed November 2018) & Gallagher JC, MacDougall C. Antibiotics Simplified – 3rd edition © Jones & Bartlett Publishing

Consideration of When to Draw Cultures vs. Start Antibiotics in the Emergency Department (ED)

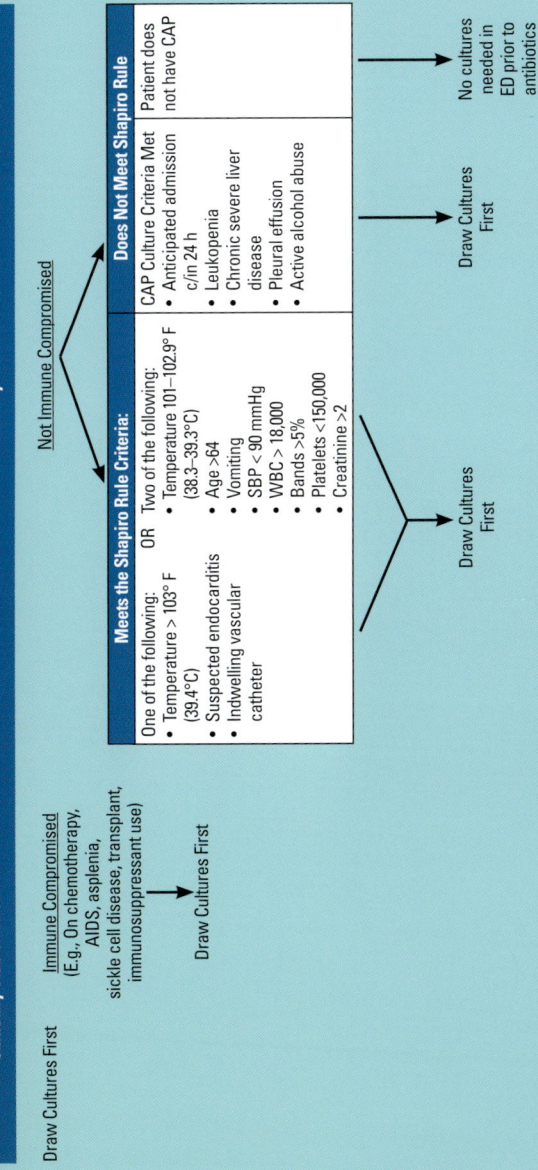

Clinically Stable Patient

Immune Compromised (E.g., On chemotherapy, AIDS, asplenia, sickle cell disease, transplant, immunosuppressant use)

Draw Cultures First

Clinically Unstable Patient

Not Immune Compromised

Meets the Shapiro Rule Criteria:

One of the following:
- Temperature > 103° F (39.4°C)
- Suspected endocarditis
- Indwelling vascular catheter

OR

Two of the following:
- Temperature 101–102.9° F (38.3–39.3°C)
- Age >64
- Vomiting
- SBP < 90 mmHg
- WBC > 18,000
- Bands >5%
- Platelets <150,000
- Creatinine >2

Draw Cultures First

Does Not Meet Shapiro Rule

CAP Culture Criteria Met
- Anticipated admission c/in 24 h
- Leukopenia
- Chronic severe liver disease
- Pleural effusion
- Active alcohol abuse

Draw Cultures First

Patient does not have CAP

No cultures needed in ED prior to antibiotics

Based on Pawlowicz A, Holland C, Zou B, Payton T, Tyndall JA, Allen B. Implementation of an evidence-based algorithm reduces blood culture overuse in an adult emergency department. Gen Int Med Clin Innov. 2016. doi:10.15761/GIMCI.1000108

CAP = Community Acquired Pneumonia; SBP = Systolic Blood Pressure; WBC = White Blood Cells

Guzman OE. Chapter 32 – Antibiotic Streamlining. Competence Assessment Tools for Health-System Pharmacies. Available at: https://www.ashp.org/-/media/store-files/p4023-sample-chapter-32.ashx. Accessed 14 November 2018.

Consider Whether to Draw a Culture (General)

Timing	Control the Source	Contamination & Colonization	Presence of Signs of Infection:
• Perform cultures before starting antibiotics if possible • Do not delay antibiotics if life-threatning: start broad & de-escalate	• Consider incision & drainage (I&D) when possible	• Signs of Possible Contamination/Colonization: Large # of epithelial cells present/growth of normal skin flora • Consider: Was the specimen collected properly	• Fever >104° F (not all patients; elderly may be hypothermic) • Systolic blood pressure < 90 mmHg (cause = dehydration/sepsis) • Heart rate > 100 bpm • Rapid breathing (>20 bpm or $PaCO_2$ < 32 mmHg if MV) • WBC 4,000 – 12,000 cells/mm^3 with possible left shift • PCT > 0.5 ng/mL

MV = Mechanical Ventilation; WBC = White Blood Cells; PCT = Procalcitonin

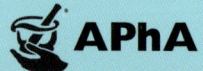

Usual Pediatric Dosages of Common Over-the-Counter (OTC) Medications

Background/Considerations

- Over-the-counter (OTC) medications may not be labeled for use in infants or young children.
- Dosages listed represent acceptable clinical practice; dosages not listed in labeling should be given under physician guidance. Doses bolded with asterisks (*) are doses recommended for that patient group, but should be given with physician guidance.
- While age-based dosing is often available, weight-based dosing is preferred when provided. It is important to determine an accurate weight. Confirm if physician has recommended a dose to double-check dosing.
- Parents should be reminded to check expiration dates on medications at home before giving medicines to children. Doses may be recommended by the pharmacy, but the caregiver may not buy the medication because they have it at home. Instruct the parent or caregiver to check the medication strength to ensure that dosing and amounts are correct.

Administration Considerations

- When recommending or dispensing a liquid medication, ensure the care provider has an appropriate measuring device and demonstrate how much medication to fill on the device. If a medication comes with a device, that device should be used.
- When giving a volume to the care provider to draw up, make sure to recommend a quantity that is easily measurable with the device being used, such as a dosing spoon or syringe. Marking on the syringe or providing a paper version may help to ensure recall of correct volume.
  - *Note: Per the Institute for Safe Medication Practices (ISMP) recommendations, devices should only have metric units as measurements.*
  - *Parents of infants may wish to administer doses in smaller portions of the full dose at a time. This ensures that the parent will be able to quantify the amount that has been given in the event that the child spits up a portion of the medication.*
- If a child does not like the taste of the medication, it may be possible to help mask the flavor by adding the medication to other liquids (e.g., juices) or semisolids (e.g., pudding). Check "Administration" section of package insert or a pediatric-specific drug reference to determine what is okay and what should be avoided.
  - *Note that adding medications to these substances may result in the child refusing to ingest the full amount of the medication, making it difficult to quantify the dose given.*
  - *If medication is added to other substances, use a small amount of the other substance. This ensures that all of the mixture (therefore, the full dose of the medication) can be administered as a small quantity. However, if the child wants more of the substance, additional amounts can be given without the drug.*
- If medication is given via a tube, please check with the care provider or patient to see if they can use regular oral syringes or need additional devices.

Cough/Cold/Allergy

The Food and Drug Administration (FDA) and American Academy of Pediatrics (AAP) have issued public health advisories strongly recommending that over-the-counter cough and cold products should not be used in infants and children less than 2 years of age. An advisory was originally issued in 2007. In 2008, voluntary removal of OTC infant products (products targeted at children less than 2 years of age) began due to safety concerns mentioned previously.

Sample Resources
Medication Safety for Children. *Arch Pediatr Adolesc Med. 2010;* 164(2):208 in JAMA Pediatrics: Advice for Patients: (http://archpedi.jamanetwork.com/article.aspx?articleid=382713).
https://www.fda.gov/forconsumers/consumerupdates/consumerupdatesenespanol/ucm291741.htm (Accessed 2018).
Dundee FD, Dundee DM, Noday DM. Pediatric Counseling and Medication Management Services: Opportunities for Community Pharmacists. *J Am Pharm Assoc.* 2002; 42: 556-567.
https://www.fda.gov/drugs/resourcesforyou/ucm133419.htm (Accessed 2018)

Prepared by Mark Botti

Pediatric Commercially Available Dosage Forms and Doses/Concentrations of Analgesics

Acetaminophen

Weight (in pounds [lb])	Dose (in milligrams [mg])	Dose (in milliliters [mL] of 160 mg/5 mL])
6 to 11	40*	1.25*
12 to 17	80*	2.5*
18 to 23	120*	3.75*
24 to 35	160	5
36 to 47	240	7.5
48 to 59	320	10
60 to 71	400	12.5
72 to 95	480	15

Doses can be given every 4 to 6 hours. Do not give more than 5 doses in 24 hours.
Maximum daily dose is 480 mg per dose up to 5 doses, or 2400 mg total daily dose.

Liquids are available as elixir grape, cherry, berry, fruit, bubble gum, cotton candy, and strawberry. Oral disintegrating tablets are available as grape, wild grape, and bubble gum flavors. Sugar free and gluten free preparations exist. Preparations come in alcohol-free and dye-free varieties.

Ibuprofen

Weight (in pounds [lb])	Dose (in milligrams [mg])
Less than 12	Not recommended
12 to 17	50*
18 to 23	75*
24 to 35	100
36 to 47	150
48 to 59	200
60 to 71	250
72 to 95	300

Doses can be given every 6 to 8 hours.
Maximum daily dose is 40 mg/kg/day up to 1200 mg/day. Maximum of 4 doses per day.
Available as an oral suspension with flavors of fruit, grape, blue-raspberry, white grape, berry, tropical punch, and bubble gum. Comes in alcohol-free, dye-free, and sugar-free varieties. Chewable tabs available in grape and orange flavors.

Medication	Dosage Forms	Doses and Concentrations of Commercially Available Products
Acetaminophen	Chewable tablets	80 mg
	Liquid	160 mg/5 mL
	Orally disintegrating tablets	80 mg, 160 mg
	Suppositories	80 mg, 160 mg, 325 mg, 650 mg
	Tablets/caplets	325 mg, 500 mg, 625 mg
Ibuprofen	Capsule/tablet	100 mg (tablet only), 200 mg
	Chewable tablets	100 mg
	Liquids	50 mg/1.25 mL, 100 mg/5 mL, 200 mg/5 mL

*Note: * = doses recommended for that patient group, but should only be given with physician guidance.*

Prepared by Mark Botti

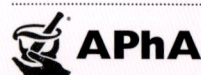

Pediatric Commercially Available Dosage Forms and Doses/Concentrations of Antihistamines

Cetirizine

Age	Dose (in milligrams [mg])	Dose (in milliliters [mL] of liquid)
<6 months	Not recommended	Not applicable
6 to 12 months	2.5 mg once daily	2.5 mg = 2.5 mL
12 to 23 months	Initial: 2.5 mg once daily. May increase to 2.5 mg twice daily	
2 to 5 years	Initial: 2.5 mg once daily. May increase to 2.5 mg twice daily or 5 mg daily	5 mg = 5 mL
≥6 years	5 to 10 mg per day as one dose or divided into 2 doses	10 mg = 10 mL

Solution and syrups available as a hydrochloride are available as a liquid preparation in grape, banana-grape, and bubble gum flavor. Solutions are often dye free, gluten free, and sugar free (verify with specific product). Chewable tablets are available as tutti-frutti, grape, and citrus.

Loratadine

Age	Dose (in milligrams [mg])	Dose (in milliliters [mL] of liquid)
<2 years	Not recommended	Not applicable
2 to 5 years	5 mg once daily	5 mL
≥6 years	10 mg once daily	10 mL

Solution and syrups available as a hydrochloride are available as liquid preparations in grape, banana-grape, and fruit flavor. Chewable tablets available as grape flavor. Oral disintegrating tablets (ODT) available as bubblegum, citrus, and fruit flavors. Solutions are often alcohol free, dye free, gluten free, and sugar free (verify with specific product).

Diphenhydramine

Age (years)	Usual dose	Max daily dose
<2	Not recommended	Not applicable
2 to 6	**6.25 to 12.5 mg***	**37.5 mg/day***
6 to 11	12.5 to 25 mg	150 mg/day
≥12	25 to 50 mg	300 mg/day

* Doses for 2 to < 4 years should be given under physician guidance.* Dose is 5 mg/kg/day divided into 3 to 4 doses as needed or every 4 to 8 hours. Do not take more than 6 doses/day. Comes in alcohol-free, dye-free, sorbitol-free, and sugar-free options. Liquids available with cherry, fruit, berry, mango, and vanilla cherry. Strips are grape flavored. Tablets available as cherry and grape flavors.

Commercially Available Products

Medication	Dosage Forms	Commercially Available Products
Cetirizine	Capsules/Dispersible Tablets	10 mg
	Chewable Tablets/Tablets	5 mg, 10 mg
	Liquid	5 mg/5 mL
Diphenhydramine	Capsules/Tablets	25 mg, 50 mg
	Chewable Tablets/Strips	12.5 mg
	Liquid	5 mg/5 mL, 12.5 mg/5 mL
Loratadine	Capsules/Tablets	10 mg
	Chewable Tablets	5 mg
	Dispersible Tablets	5 mg, 10 mg
	Liquids	5 mg/5 mL

Note: Doses bolded with asterisks (*) are recommended for that patient group, but should only be given with physician guidance.

Prepared by Mark Botti

Pediatric Commercially Available Dosage Forms and Doses for Antiflatulents

Simethicone		
Age	**Dose (in milligrams [mg])**	**Dose (in milliliters [mL] of liquid)**
< 2 years	20	0.3
2 to 12 years	40	0.6
> 12 years	40–125; may give single dose of 500 mg; do not exceed 500 mg per day	Consider chewable tabs

Administer up to 4 times per day with meals.
Chewable tabs available in cherry crème, cool mint, peppermint, and peppermint crème. Strips available in cinnamon and peppermint. Suspension available in fruit and vanilla. Some formulations come alcohol free, dye free, and/or saccharin free.

Medication	**Dosage Forms**	**Doses/Concentrations Available**
Simethicone	Capsule	125 mg, 180 mg
	Chewable tablets	80 mg, 125 mg
	Liquids	20 mg/0.3 mL
	Strips	40 mg, 62.5 mg

Pediatric Measurements

Measuring Device	**Size**	**Measure to Nearest**	**Potential Alternative Doses**
Oral syringe*	1 mL	0.02 mL	N/A
	3 mL	0.1 mL	1.25 mL Using ¼ tsp mark
	5 mL	0.2 mL	1.25 mL, 2.5 mL, 3.75 mL Using ¼, ½, ¾ tsp marks
	10 mL	0.2 mL	2.5 mL, 7.5 mL Using ½, 1½ tsp marks
Dosing spoon	10 mL	1 mL	1.25 mL, 2.5 mL, 3.75 mL, 7.5 mL ¼, ½, ¾, 1½ tsp marks
Dosing cup	Variable	Check dosing cup	Variable

Note: * = ISMP (Institute for Safe Medication Practices) only recommends use of oral syringes with metric doses. Other nonmetric syringes not recommended; N/A = not applicable.

Prepared by Mark Botti

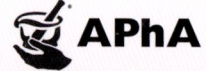

Inappropriate Medications in Older Adults

BEERS CRITERIA
The Beers Criteria for Potentially Inappropriate Medication Use in Older Adults was originally published in 1991. Subsequent updates occurred in 1997, 2003, and 2012. The most recent updated edition was released in 2015.[1] This update removes drugs no longer available, adds new drugs, and adds an expanded list of conditions considered. The new update also uses an evidence-based approach in developing the guidelines and a rating system for each criterion.

KEY POINTS
- The criteria are not meant to substitute for professional, clinical judgment, and therapy should be individualized for each patient.
- The criteria are meant to "inform clinical decision making, research, training, and policy to improve the quality and safety of prescribing medications for older adults."[1]
- The Screening Tool of Older Persons' Potentially Inappropriate Prescriptions and Screening Tool to Alert Doctors to the Right Treatment (STOPP/START criteria) should be used in a complementary manner to the Beers Criteria.[3]

ORGANIZATION/RESOURCE
The American Geriatrics Society (AGS) has a printable pocket card available for download on the organization's website: *http://www.geriatricscareonline.org/ProductAbstract/beers-pocket-card/PC001* (Accessed November 2018). The card organizes content from the updated Beers Criteria in extensive tables:

- Table 2: 2015 AGS Beers Criteria for Potentially Inappropriate Medication Use in Older Adults by ***Organ System/ Therapeutic Category/Drug(s)***
- Table 3: 2015 AGS Beers Criteria for Potentially Inappropriate Medication Use in Older Adults Due to ***Drug-Disease or Drug-Syndrome Interactions That May Exacerbate the Disease or Syndrome***
- Table 4: Medications to Be Used with Caution
- Table 5: Clinically Important Non-anti-infective Drug-Drug Interactions
- Table 6: Non-anti-infective Medications to Avoid or Dosage Adjustments Based on Kidney Function

OTHER INFORMATION
Most adverse drug events in older adults are attributed to a small number of medications. Four medication classes were found in a recent study to be responsible for the most adverse effects in adults: warfarin, insulin, oral antiplatelet agents, and oral hypoglycemic agents.[2,3] Close monitoring of these medication classes should be employed to reduce patient risk.

REFERENCES
1. American Geriatrics Society 2015 Beers Criteria Update Panel. American Geriatrics Society Updated Beers Criteria for Potentially Inappropriate Medication Use in Older Adults. *J Am Geriatr Soc*, 2015. DOI: 10.1111/jgs.13702.
2. O'Mahony D, O'Sullivan D, Byrne S, et al. STOPP/START criteria for potentially inappropriate prescribing in older people: Version 2. *Age & Ageing* 2015; 44:213–18.
3. Budnitz DS, Lovegrove MC, Shehab N, Richards CL. Emergency hospitalizations for adverse drug events in older Americans. *N Engl J Med*, 2011. 365: 2002–12.

Inappropriate Medications in Older Adults *(continued)*

Ten Medications to Avoid in Older Adults	Additional Information
1. **Nonsteroidal Anti-Inflammatory Drugs (NSAIDs)**	• Avoid due to risk of indigestion, ulcers, & bleeding. • Shorter-acting versions are considered a safer choice. • These medications should not be taken with other medications that increase risk of bleeding.
2. **Certain Diabetes Drugs**	• Certain diabetes medications, such as glyburide may result in hypoglycemic episodes in older adults.
3. **Certain Cardiovascular Drugs**	• Digoxin: avoid doses > 0.125 mg, which can result in toxicity. • Certain blood pressure medications may increase risk of orthostatic hypotension or bradycardia. • Aspirin: evidence versus benefit in adults 80 years of age & older. • Prasugrel: increased caution over the age of 75. • Other: warfarin, angiotensin-converting-enzyme inhibitors (ACEI); alpha-1 blockers; amiodarone; nifedipine; & others.
4. **Muscle Relaxants**	• Muscle relaxants can cause sedation, increased confusion, fall risk, constipation, dry mouth & urinary retention. • Examples include cyclobenzaprine & methocarbamol.
5. **Medications for Anxiety/ Insomnia**	• Medications for anxiety and insomnia can increase risk of falls & confusion.
6. **Certain Anticholinergic Drugs**	• Anticholinergic drugs may result in confusion, constipation, urinary retention, blurred vision, & hypotension. • Examples may include certain antidepressants, certain anti-Parkinson drugs, dicyclomine, & oxybutynin.
7. **Meperidine**	• This medication may cause risk of confusion & seizures.
8. **Certain Antihistamine Medications**	• Certain antihistamines may result in confusion, constipation, urinary retention, blurred vision, & dry mouth.
9. **Antipsychotics** (if not treated for psychosis)	• Haloperidol, risperidone, and quetiapine are antipsychotic medications that may result in increased risk of stroke as well as other side effects such as tremors & increased fall risk.
10. **Estrogens**	• Estrogens increase older adults' risk for clots & dementia.

Reference: Information adapted from Ten Medications Older Adults Should Avoid or Use with Caution. Healthinaging.org: Trusted Information. Better Care by the American Geriatrics Foundation for Health in Aging. Full content available at: http://www.healthinaging.org/files/documents/tipsheets/meds_to_avoid.pdf (Accessed November 2018).

Brief Overview of STOPP/START Criteria
- **STOPP** (screening tool of older people's prescriptions): 80 clinically significant criteria for potentially inappropriate medication use (drug and disease interactions, therapeutic duplication)
- **START** (screening tool to alert to right treatment): 34 common disease states in older adults where medications are indicated (evidence based)
- Organized as analgesic, cardiovascular, central nervous system, endocrine, gastrointestinal, respiratory, and urinary tract drugs.

Prepared by Jeanine P. Abrons

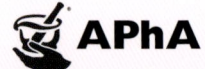

Pregnancy and Lactation Resources

Name of Resource	How to Access	Description
LactMed (Drugs and Lactation Database)	http://toxnet.nlm. nih.gov/newtoxnet/ lactmed.htm (Accessed November 2018)	• From the website: "The LactMed® database contains information on drugs and other chemicals to which breastfeeding mothers may be exposed." • Components listed: Levels anticipated; effects in breastfed infants; effects on lactation and breast milk; alternatives to consider; references • Updated monthly
Briggs' Drugs in Pregnancy and Lactation, Ninth Edition	Wolters Kluwer Health/Lippincott Williams and Wilkins Textbook; Partial (preview) version available as free download at iTunes Store	• Summarizes known/possible side effects of medications in pregnancy and possibility of passage through breast milk when nursing; A to Z searchable index • Includes: Generic name; pharmacological class; risk factor; fetal risk summary; breast feeding summary; references
Medication and a Mother's Milk	Overview: http:// www.medsmilk.com (Accessed November 2018)	• Includes recommendations by the American Academy of Pediatrics • Also includes drug name/generic name; uses; drug monograph (understood knowledge of the drug; ability to enter milk; time dependent concentration; other clinically relevant information); pregnancy risk category; lactation risk category; theoretical/relative infant dose; adult/pediatric concerns; drug interactions; alternatives; pharmacokinetic/pharmacodynamics information
Infant Risk Center	http://www.infantrisk. com (Accessed November 2018)	• Provided by Texas Tech University Health Sciences Center • Tabs on Pregnancy and Breastfeeding under "Trending Topics" • Provides general information on select topics related to pregnancy and breastfeeding

Consult multiple resources, as recommendations may differ.

Known Teratogens
Alcohol; angiotensin-converting-enzyme inhibitors (ACEI); angiotensin receptor blockers (ARBs); carbamazepine; cocaine; coumarin anticoagulants; diethylstilbestrol (DES); methotrexate; phenytoin; isotretinoin; lithium; misoprostol; statins; tetracyclines; thalidomide; valproate

Reference: Walters Burkey B, Holmes AP. Evaluating Medication Use in Pregnancy and Lactation: What Every Pharmacist Should Know. *J Pediatr Pharmacol Ther.* 2013; 18(3): 247–58.

Prepared by Jeanine P. Abrons

Pregnancy Risk Classifications

Risk Classification	Description		
Food and Drug Administration (FDA) Drug Classification System	**Current Labeling**		**New Labeling (effective June 2015)**
	8.1 Pregnancy	→	8.1 Pregnancy (includes Labor and Delivery)
	8.2 Labor and Delivery	→	Merged Into 8.1 Pregnancy
	8.3 Nursing Mothers	→	8.2 Lactation (includes Nursing Mothers)
			NEW 8.3 Females and Males Reproductive Potential
	• The FDA published the "Content and Format of Labeling for Human Prescription Drug and Biological Products; Requirements for Pregnancy and Lactation Labeling" (also known as the Pregnancy and Lactation Labeling Rule) [PLLR] in 2014. The PLLR requires changes to content/format of prescription labeling to assist providers in determining risk versus benefit for pregnant and nursing. The law requires the label to be updated when content becomes outdated. The change went into effect June 30, 2015. Medications approved prior to June 29, 2001, are not subject to the new rule, but must have the letter category removed by June 29, 2018.		
Teratogen Information System (TERIS)	• Describes risk as "unlikely," "none or minimal risk," "small to moderate," "moderate to high risk," or "risk undetermined." • Further information available at http://depts.washington.edu/terisweb/teris/ (Accessed November 2018).		

Reference: http://www.fda.gov/Drugs/DevelopmentApprovalProcess/DevelopmentResources/Labeling/ucm093307.htm (November 2018).

Prepared by Jeanine P. Abrons

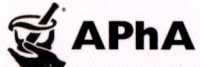

Safe and Unsafe Use of OTC Medications during Pregnancy

Common Conditions	UNSAFE OTC Treatments during Pregnancy: Trimester UNSAFE to Use	SAFE OTC Treatments during Pregnancy: Trimester SAFE to Use
Allergic Rhinitis	• Fexofenadine**(Allegra®): 1st	• **Chlorpheniramine; DOC:** all trimesters • Cetirizine (Zyrtec®): 2nd, 3rd • Loratadine (Claritin®): 2nd, 3rd
Congestion	• Phenylephrine: 1st • Pseudoephedrine: 1st	• Nasal saline sprays: all trimesters • Adhesive nasal strips: all trimesters • Use of a humidifier: all trimesters
Cough	• Guaifenesin: 1st • Codeine: all trimesters (especially 1st, 3rd)	• Dextromethorphan*: all trimesters
Pain, Fever, and Headache	• Aspirin: do not use • Ibuprofen: 3rd • Naproxen: 3rd • Aspirin/acetaminophen/caffeine (Excedrin®): do not use	• **Acetaminophen*; DOC:** all trimesters
Nausea	• Meclizine**: caution in all	• Vitamin B6^: all trimesters • Doxylamine: all trimesters • Ginger^: all trimesters
Fungal Infections and Dermatitis	• Clotrimazole: 2nd, 3rd • Miconazole: 2nd, 3rd • Tioconazole**: 2nd, 3rd	• Topical antifungals: all trimesters • Butoconazole: 2nd, 3rd • Hydrocortisone*: all trimesters
Heartburn	• Antacids: avoid doses with high amounts of calcium and aluminum	• **Calcium carbonate; DOC:** all trimesters • Omeprazole (Prilosec®): all trimesters • Antacids with Al-, Ca^{2+}, Mg^{2+}: all trimesters • Ranitidine (Zantac®) > cimetidine for chronic use: all trimesters • Famotidine (Pepcid®)**: All trimesters
Diarrhea	• Loperamide** (Imodium®): 1st • Bismuth subsalicylate (Pepto-Bismol®): do not use	• **Kaolin and pectin** (Kaopectate®); DOC:** all trimesters
Constipation	• Mineral oil: do not use • Castor oil: do not use	• **Polyethylene glycol 3350** (Miralax®); DOC:** all trimesters
Dermatologic Disorders/Acne	• Salicylic acid (BHA) > 2%: do not use • Retinoids/retinol: do not use	• Salicylic acid (BHA) $\leq$ 2%: all trimesters • Benzoyl peroxide: all trimesters • Glycolic acid (AHA): all trimesters

Notes: DOC = drug of choice; PPI = proton pump inhibitors.

* = recommend lowest strength for shortest time possible; ** = limited human data; ^ = herbal/vitamin supplement.

This table is for general information. Always have patients discuss medications and supplements with an obstetrician. Generally, medications under "UNSAFE" have specifically been stated in literature to use with caution, to avoid in certain trimesters, to have limited human data, or to have better alternatives. Medications under "SAFE" are either DOCs, have not been cautioned for use, or do not have specific restrictions documented in literature.

References: (Accessed November 2018)
American Academy of Family Physicians website: *http://www.aafp.org/afp/2014/1015/p548.html#afp20141015p548-t3*
CDC website. *http://www.cdc.gov/pregnancy/meds/treatingfortwo/facts.html*
American Pregnancy Association website: *http://americanpregnancy.org/pregnancy-complications/cough-cold-during-pregnancy*

Prepared by Brittany Hayes; updated by Jeanine P. Abrons

Immunization Schedule for Children and Adults Ages 18 Years or Younger

Vaccine	Dose/Recommended Ages for All Children	Recommended Ages for Catch-up Immunization	Other/Notes
Hepatitis B (HepB)	• 1st dose: Birth • 2nd dose: 1 month–2 months • 3rd dose: 6–8 months	• 4 months–18 years • Adolescents 11–15 years may use alternative 2-dose schedule, with at least 4 months between doses	• Minimum age: birth (monovalent HepB vaccine only)—Timing of dosing depends on weight of infant and whether mom is HBsAg(-), (+), or status is unknown—see footnotes for guidance** • Minimum interval between doses 1 & 2 = 4 weeks • Minimum interval between doses 2 & 3 = 8 weeks (16 weeks after 1st dose) • Minimum age for final dose = 24 weeks
Rotavirus (RV) RV$_1$ (2-dose series) RV$_5$ (3-dose series)	• 1st dose (both): 2 months • 2nd dose (both): 4 months • 3rd dose (RV$_5$ only): 6 months	• 14 weeks 6 days = max age for 1st dose • 8 months = max age for final dose	• Minimum age 6 weeks for both vaccines • If vaccine product is unknown, administer 3 doses • Rotarix: 2-dose series at 2 & 4 months • RotaTeq: 3-dose series at 2, 4, & 6 months
Diphtheria, tetanus, & acellular pertussis (DTaP)	• 1st dose: 2 months • 2nd dose: 4 months • 3rd dose: 6 months • 4th dose: 15 thru 18 months • 5th dose: 4 to 6 years	• 9 months–4 years • 5th dose not needed if 4th dose given at ≥ age 4	• Minimum age: 6 weeks (4 years for Kinrix or Quadracel) • DTaP: < 7 years • Minimum interval between doses 1 & 2; 2 & 3 = 4 weeks • Minimum interval between doses 3 & 4; 4 & 5 = 6 months • 5-dose series at 2, 4, 6, 15–18 months, & 4–6 years
Haemophilus influenza type b (Hib)	• 1st dose: 2 months • 2nd dose: 4 months • 3rd dose*: 6 months or see booster dose • Booster dose*: Age 12–15 months	• Age impacted by timing of 1st dose & formulation; typical spacing of doses varies from 4–8 weeks	• Minimum age = 6 weeks for PCV13 & 2 years for PPSV23 • *For ActHIB, Hiberix, or Pentacel only: 4-dose series at 2, 4, 6, & 12–15 months • PedvaxHIB = 3-dose series at 2, 4, & 12–15 months • Dosing for certain high-risk groups: age 12–59 months & 5–18 years • See footnotes guidance at cdc.gov** • For minimum intervals between doses, refer to cdc.gov
Pneumococcal conjugate (PCV13)	• 1st dose: 2 months • 2nd dose: 4 months • 3rd dose: 6 months • 4th dose: 12–15 months	• 24–59 months (administer 1 dose to healthy children not completely vaccinated)	• Minimum age = 6 weeks • For certain high-risk groups: ages 2–5 & 6–18 years • For minimum intervals between doses. refer to cdc.gov **

Note: * = 3 dose and 4 dose series available; timing of a booster dose depends on whether child received primary series in the first year of life; http://www.immunize.org/askexperts/experts_hib.asp; https://www.cdc.gov/vaccines/hcp/vis/vis-statements/hib.html; ** = https://www.cdc.gov/vaccines/schedules/hcp/child-adolescent.html (Accessed November 2018)

Prepared by Jeanine P. Abrons and Elisha Andreas

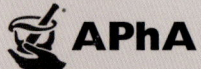

Vaccine	Dose/Recommended Ages for All Children	Information Related to Catch-up Immunization/Other Notes
Serogroup A,C,W, Y meningococcal vaccine*	• 1st dose of Menactra or Menveo: 11–12 years • 2nd dose or booster of Menactra or Menveo 16 years	• Minimum age: 2 months (Menveo), 9 months (Menactra) • Age 13–15 years: 1 dose now & booster at age 16–18 years. Minimum interval 8 weeks • Age 16–18 years: 1 dose • Menactra should be given either before or at the same time as DTaP • Different from the serogroup B vaccine (min age: 10 years [Bexsero, Trumenba]. Clinical discretion: Adolescents not at ↑ risk for meningococcal B infection who want the vaccine & 16–23 years (preferred age 16–18 years).** • Minimum interval between dose 1 & 2 = 8 weeks
Tetanus, diphtheria, & acellular pertussis (Tdap)	• 1st dose: 11–12 years	• Not fully immunized with DTaP: 1 dose of Tdap after age 7; if more doses needed use tetanus & diphtheria (Td) • Children 7–10 years dose as catch-up: additional dose at 11–12 • 11–18 years: give 1st dose then Td booster every 10 years • Tdap minimum age = 10 years • May be administered regardless of the interval since last tetanus/diphtheria containing vaccine • Administer 1 dose in pregnancy (preferably between weeks 27–36) • Children age ≥ 7 years who are not fully immunized with DTaP should receive Tdap vaccine as 1 dose in catch-up series, adolescent Tdap at age 11–12 may be given • Persons age 11–18 who have not gotten Tdap vaccine should receive a dose, followed by tetanus & diphtheria booster dose every 10 years after. For inadvertent doses of DTaP: see CDC website**
Human papillomavirus	• Routine vaccination for ages 11–12, may start at age 9: Give series on schedule of 0, 6–12 months; can start at age 9 • Administer thru age 18 • 1st dose before age 15: 2 doses on schedule of 0, 6–12 months; minimum interval = 5 months • 1st dose at or after age 15: 3 doses on schedule of 0, 1–2, 6 months	• Vaccine dose administered at shorter intervals than minimum 2-dose schedule interval • Minimum age of 9 for routine/catch-up doses • Number of recommended doses based on age of administration of 1st dose • If vaccine administered on shorter interval than recommended, re-administer after minimum interval has been met • Age 15 years or older at initiation: 3-dose series minimum intervals: 4 weeks between 1st & 2nd dose; 12 weeks between 2nd & 3rd dose; 5 months between 1st & 3rd dose • 12 weeks between 2nd & 3rd; 5 months between 1st & 3rd dose • See CDC site for special populations**

Note: *For meningococcal B vaccination pneumococcal polysaccharide (PPSV23), see CDC website for use in high-risk conditions & other persons at increased risk of disease. ** = https://www.cdc.gov/vaccines/schedules/hcp/child-adolescent.html (Accessed November 2018).

Prepared by Jeanine P. Abrons and Elisha Andreas

Immunizations by Age for First Year of Life

Age	Immunizations to Be Given During Normal Dosing Schedule	Needle Length/Injection Site
Birth	• Hepatitis B*	Intramuscular: 5/8"; anterolateral thigh muscle; use 22- to 25-gauge needle
1 month	• Hepatitis B (or month 2)*	Subcutaneous: 5/8" fatty tissue over anterolateral thigh muscle; use 23- to 25-gauge needle Intramuscular: 1" in anterolateral thigh muscle; use 22- to 25-gauge needle
2 months	• Diphtheria, tetanus, & acellular pertussis (DTaP < 7 years)* • Hepatitis B (or month 1) (2nd dose if not given at month 1)* • Haemophilus influenza type b (1st dose)* • Inactivated poliovirus (IPV < 18 years) (1st dose)	• Pneumococcal conjugate (PCV13) (1st dose)* • Rotavirus (1st dose)**
4 months	• Rotavirus (2nd dose)** • Diphtheria, tetanus, & acellular pertussis (DTaP < 7 years)* • Haemophilus influenza type b (2nd dose)* • Pneumococcal conjugate (PCV13) (2nd dose)*	• Inactivated poliovirus (IPV < 18 years) (2nd dose)* • Catch-up immunization potential: hepatitis B*
6 months	• Diphtheria, tetanus, & acellular pertussis (DTaP < 7 years)* • Haemophilus influenza type b (if 3 or 4 dose series)* • Hepatitis B (potentially) 3rd dose may be given 6 months on* • Inactivated poliovirus (IPV < 18 years) (potentially) 3rd dose may be given 6 months on†	• Influenza (annually, potential)** • Pneumococcal conjugate (PCV13) (3rd dose)* • Rotavirus (if 3-dose series)**
9 months	• Hepatitis B (potentially) If 3rd dose not already given* • Inactivated poliovirus (IPV < 18 years) (potentially) If 3rd dose not already given† • Influenza (annually; potential)**	• Catch-up immunization potential: diphtheria, tetanus, & acellular pertussis (DTaP < 7 years)*, haemophilus* influenza type b; pneumococcal conjugate (PCV13)* • Certain high-risk groups: measles, mumps, rubella (MMR)***
12 months	• Hepatitis B (potentially) If 3rd dose not already given* • Haemophilus influenza type b (if 3 or 4 dose series)* • Inactivated poliovirus (IPV < 18 years) (potentially) If 3rd dose not already given† • Influenza (annually; potential)** • Measles, mumps, rubella (MMR)***	• Hepatitis A (potentially)* • Pneumococcal conjugate (PCV13) (potentially 4th dose)* • Varicella (potentially 1st dose)*** • Catch-up immunization potential: diphtheria, tetanus, & acellular pertussis (DTaP < 7 years)*

Notes: * = dose or route of administration & dose dependent upon product; *** = Dose subcutaneously of 0.5 mL; + = Dose intramuscularly (IM) or subcutaneously of 0.5 mL. References: with https://www.cdc.gov/vaccines/schedules/hcp/imz/child-adolescent-shell.html#f10; immunize.org (Accessed 2018)

Prepared by Jeanine P. Abrons and Elisha Andreas

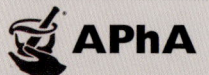

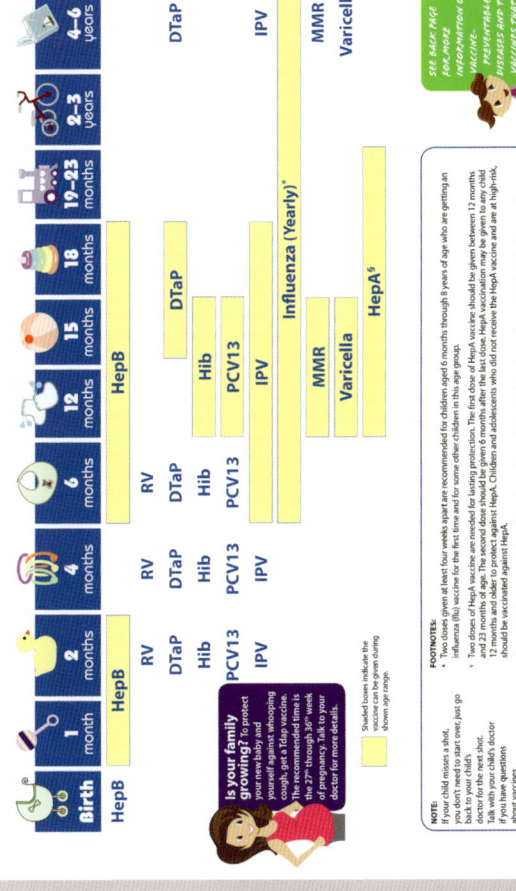

2018 Recommended Immunizations for Children from Birth Through 6 Years Old

	Birth	1 month	2 months	4 months	6 months	12 months	15 months	18 months	19–23 months	2–3 years	4–6 years
HepB	HepB	HepB				HepB					
RV			RV	RV	RV						
DTaP			DTaP	DTaP	DTaP		DTaP				DTaP
Hib			Hib	Hib	Hib	Hib					
PCV13			PCV13	PCV13	PCV13	PCV13					
IPV			IPV	IPV	IPV	IPV					IPV
Influenza						Influenza (Yearly)*					
MMR						MMR					MMR
Varicella						Varicella					Varicella
HepA						HepA⁵					

Shaded boxes indicate the vaccine can be given during shown age range.

Is your family growing? To protect your new baby and yourself against whooping cough, get a Tdap vaccine. The recommended time is the 27th through 36th week of pregnancy. Talk to your doctor for more details.

NOTE:
If your child misses a shot, you don't need to start over, just go back to your child's doctor for the next shot. Talk with your child's doctor if you have questions about vaccines.

FOOTNOTES:
* Two doses given at least four weeks apart are recommended for children aged 6 months through 8 years of age who are getting an influenza (flu) vaccine for the first time and for some other children in this age group.

⁵ Two doses of HepA vaccine are needed for lasting protection. The first dose of HepA vaccine should be given between 12 months and 23 months of age. The second dose should be given 6 months after the last dose. HepA vaccination may be given to any child 12 months and older to protect against HepA. Children and adolescents who did not receive the HepA vaccine and are at high-risk, should be vaccinated against HepA.

If your child has any medical conditions that put him at risk for infection or is traveling outside the United States, talk to your child's doctor about additional vaccines that he may need.

SEE BACK PAGE FOR MORE INFORMATION ON VACCINE-PREVENTABLE DISEASES AND THE VACCINES THAT PREVENT THEM.

For more information, call toll free
1-800-CDC-INFO (1-800-232-4636)
or visit
www.cdc.gov/vaccines/parents

U.S. Department of Health and Human Services
Centers for Disease Control and Prevention

CDC

AMERICAN ACADEMY OF FAMILY PHYSICIANS
STRONG MEDICINE FOR AMERICA

American Academy of Pediatrics
DEDICATED TO THE HEALTH OF ALL CHILDREN®

Content source: National Center for Immunization and Respiratory Diseases.
Reference: https://www.cdc.gov/vaccines/parents/downloads/parent-ver-sch-0-6yrs.pdf [Accessed November 2018]

Travel Immunization and Travel Health Card

	Tourists	Long-term travelers & expatriates	VRFs[a]	Humanitarian travelers	Rural travelers	Travelers to high altitude (>8000 ft = 2500 m)	Travelers with chronic illnesses[1,4]	Pregnant travelers[6]	Pediatric travelers[6]	Last-minute travelers	Immuno-compromised travelers[b,4]
IMMUNIZATIONS											
Age-appropriate routine vaccines[1,2]											
Hepatitis A[3]						2 doses					
Hepatitis B[4]						3 doses					
Typhoid[5]					1 injectable dose or 4 oral doses						
Yellow fever[6]						1 dose					
Rabies (preexposure)[7]		3 doses							3 doses		
Japanese encephalitis[8]											
Meningococcal[9]		2 doses		1 or more doses depending on indication							
Cholera[10]				1 dose							
TB testing[11]											
OTHER											
Malaria chemoprophylaxis[12]											
Travelers' diarrhea self-treatment[13]											
Acetazolamide[14]											

Legend:
- Consider for all persons in this category
- Consider if certain geographical or behavioral risk factors are present and potential benefits outweigh risks
- Generally not recommended
- No recommendation

a. Travelers who are visiting friends and/or relatives (VFRs) (generally defined as those returning to a home country).
b. Recommendations vary based on degree and type of immune system compromise. Severely immunocompromised patients include HIV+ with CD4 <200/mm³, asplenia, transplant recipients.

Developed by the APhA-APPM Immunizing Pharmacists Special Interest Group (SIG) Travel Committee

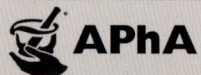

Travel Immunization and Travel Health Card *(continued)*

	Vaccination	Indication or When to Consider/Description
1	ROUTINE VACCINATIONS	Ensure that all patients are up-to-date on routine adult or age-appropriate pediatric vaccines. May include influenza (yearly), tetanus/diphtheria/pertussis, varicella, HPV, zoster, MMR, pneumococcal, polio, hepatitis A, hepatitis B, meningococcal, & *Haemophilus influenza* type B. Routine vaccines with travel-specific indications or considerations are discussed below. Use of CDC catch-up immunization schedule may be necessary for pediatric patients who are un/undervaccinated.
2	TETANUS-CONTAINING VACCINATIONS	For all patients who do not have documentation of at least one dose within the last 10 years. Indicated for adults every 10 years following final pediatric dose at 11–12 years. Adults should receive a single dose of Tdap then Td every 10 years.
3	HEPATITIS A VACCINATION	For all susceptible persons traveling to or working in countries that have high or intermediate rates of hepatitis A before traveling. • Children 6–11 months should be protected when traveling outside the United States to an area of risk. ○ This vaccine should be in addition to the routine recommended 2-dose schedule. • Persons ages ≥ 1 year can receive the age-appropriate dose of hepatitis A vaccine. • The initial dose of vaccine along with IM immune globulin at a separate injection site is recommended for the following travelers who are planning to depart to an area of risk in < 2 weeks: Adults ages > 40 years, immunocompromised people, people with chronic liver disease, people with other chronic medical conditions. • Persons who are unable to receive the hepatitis A vaccine, including those who are allergic to the vaccine & children < 6 months, should receive a single dose of immune globulin, which provides up to 2 months of protection.

4	HEPATITIS B VACCINATION	For all unvaccinated people traveling to areas with intermediate to high prevalence of chronic hepatitis B.
		• Vaccination to prevent hepatitis B may be considered for all international travelers, regardless of destination, depending on the traveler's behavioral risk or chronic disease diagnosis.
		• Hepatitis B vaccination should begin ≥ 6 months before travel so full vaccine series can be completed before departure.
		  ○ An accelerated dosing schedule may be considered for patients at significant risk if there is not sufficient time to complete the series prior to departure.
		  ○ For lower risk patients, 1 or 2 doses may be administered prior to departure, but optimal protection is reliable only after complete series.
		• Adult patients receiving hemodialysis or with other immunocompromising conditions: consult package insert for differences in dosing.

5	TYPHOID VACCINE	For all patients traveling to increased risk areas of exposure to *Salmonella* Typhi. Formulation choice based on age, patient preference, & departure time. • Typhim-Vi: Inactivated polysaccharide vaccine approved for patients ages ≥ 2 years. Single IM dose should be administered ≥ 2 weeks prior to possible exposure for optimal protection, but may be considered for last-minute travelers. May be re-dosed every 2 years if at continued risk. • Vivotif: Live-attenuated oral vaccine approved for patients ages > 6 years. All 4 oral capsules, taken 1 capsule every other day, should be taken for optimal protection & completed 1 week prior to possible exposure. May be re-dosed every 5 years if at continued risk.
6	YELLOW FEVER VACCINE	Those traveling to or through yellow fever endemic area or when vaccination is necessary for legal reasons. Consult CDC for destination specific recommendations at http://wwwnc.cdc.gov/travel/destinations/list. • Yellow fever vaccine should be avoided in children < 6 months, those allergic to gelatin, latex, or egg proteins, or in severely immunocompromised. HIV infection with CD4 count 200 to 499/mm³ is a precaution for yellow fever vaccine. (May offer vaccine instead of vaccination when benefit does not outweigh risk.) • Consider risk-benefit, especially in patients ≥ 60 years old receiving first dose of yellow fever vaccine. • Women who are pregnant should only be vaccinated if travel to a yellow fever endemic area is unavoidable & benefits of vaccination outweigh risks. • WHO/CDC now consider a single dose to be protective for life. Country-specific regulations may still require dosing every 10 years.

Travel Immunization and Travel Health Card *(continued)*

	Vaccination	Indication or When to Consider/Description
7	**PREEXPOSURE RABIES VACCINATION**	For those who plan to or may come in contact with potentially rabid animals (e.g., rabies field workers, veterinarians, wildlife biologists, etc.) &/or with prolonged travel or shorter stays in high-risk areas (e.g., epidemic outbreaks) or with extensive outdoor stays. • Preexposure vaccination simplifies postexposure regimen but does not eliminate need for vaccination after exposure. • Rabies vaccine should not be given if time does not permit completion of series prior to departure.
8	**JAPANESE ENCEPHALITIS (JE) VACCINE**	For long-term & recurrent travelers who plan to spend ≥ 1 month in endemic areas (Asia & parts of Western Pacific) during JE virus transmission season or expatriates traveling to rural or agricultural areas during high-risk period of JE virus transmission. • May consider for short-term travelers (< 1 month) to endemic areas if during JE virus transmission season/outside an urban area & activities will increase risk of JE virus exposure; traveling to area with ongoing JE outbreak or specific destination unknown or during peak transmission season (usually May-Dec, but may differ based on country, activities, or duration of travel). • Not recommended for short-term travelers whose visits will be restricted to urban areas or times outside a well-defined JE virus transmission season.
9	**MENINGOCOCCAL VACCINATION**	For patients who travel to/live in countries where meningococcal disease is hyperendemic or epidemic, including Sub-Saharan Africa meningitis belt during dry season (Dec–June). Vaccination within 3 years before travel required for entry into Saudi Arabia traveling to Mecca during Hajj & Umrah pilgrimages. • Advisories for travelers to other at-risk countries are issued when epidemics are recognized. • Administer single dose of MenACWY vaccine, revaccinate with MenACWY vaccine every 5 years if increased risk for infection remains. • MenB vaccine not recommended due to meningococcal disease in these countries generally not being caused by serogroup B. • Infants/children who received Hib-MenCY-TT are not protected against serogroups A & W; should receive quadrivalent vaccine before travel to high endemic areas. • Children who received last dose at < 7 years of age should receive an additional dose of MenACWY 3 years after last dose. • Dosing schedule & number of doses dependent on age & product administered: consult package insert.
10	**CHOLERA**	Cholera: consider only for adult patients from the United States to areas of active cholera transmission. Is an oral live attenuated vaccine. • Active cholera transmission is defined as area within a country with endemic or epidemic cholera caused by *V. cholerae* O1 & has had activity within the last year. Does not include areas of rare imported or sporadic cases. • Approved for adults 18–64 years of age. Single dose, must be administered 10 days prior to potential exposure. • No data exist on safety and efficacy in pregnant or breastfeeding women & immunocompromised patients. • Not recommended for travelers not visiting areas of active cholera transmission. Pregnant women and clinician must consider risks associated with travel to active cholera area. • Should not be given to patients who have taken antibiotics (oral or parenteral) in preceding 14 days. • If chloroquine is indicated, chloroquine must be started > 10 days after cholera vaccination. • Buffer of cholera vaccine may interfere with enteric coated Ty21a (Vivotif), taking first Ty21a dose > 8 hours after cholera vaccine might ↓ potential interference. • May shed virus in stool for ≥ 7 days; potentially may transmit to close contacts. • Requires special mixing (with supplied buffer) & consumed by patient within 15 minutes after reconstitution. Follow medical waste disposal procedures. • Patients must avoid eating or drinking 60 minutes before and after ingestion of cholera vaccine.

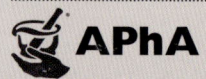

Travel Immunization and Travel Health Card *(continued)*

	Vaccination	Indication or When to Consider/Description
11	TB TESTING	Only for patients at increased risk of exposure during travel including healthcare workers, those who will have contact with prison or homeless populations, & expatriates to countries with high TB prevalence. • Two-step tuberculin skin testing (TST) should be given prior to travel (2nd test 1–3 weeks after 1st) with repeat testing q 6–12 months during possible exposure period & 8–12 weeks after return. • Alternative test: interferon-gamma release assays (IGRA) (is more specific in patients who have received BCG vaccines); may also be used if time before departure is too short for two-step TST. • TST may also be considered for VFR patients to document status prior to travel, which can aid in interpretation of future positive tests.
12	MALARIA CHEMO-PROPHYLAXIS	In combination with mosquito avoidance for all travelers to areas where malaria transmission occurs. Assess exact itinerary to determine risk for exposure & other specific factors in choice of chemoprophylaxis regimen. • Chloroquine & primaquine usefulness is limited to Central America; resistance exists in all other areas. • Avoid mefloquine in parts of South East Asia (e.g., Thailand) due to resistance. • Avoid mefloquine in patients with personal or family history of psychiatric diagnosis including depression & anxiety. • Avoid primaquine in patients who do not have documented normal G6PD levels due to risk of death due to hemolysis in deficient patients.

13	STAND-BY EMERGENCY SELF-TREATMENT OF TRAVELERS' DIARRHEA (TD)	For all travelers to developing countries.
		• First-line antibiotics include ciprofloxacin, levofloxacin, & azithromycin.
		  ○ Avoid fluoroquinolones with travel to SE Asia (resistant strains of *Camphylobacter* prevalent (e.g., Thailand))
		  ○ Antimotility agents (e.g., bismuth subsalicylate & loperimide) may be recommended as adjunct symptomatic therapy.
		• Prophylactic antibiotics not recommended except in high-risk travelers (e.g., immunocompromised). Alternate SBET antibiotics considered + prophylaxis in then.

14	ACETAZOLAMIDE ALTITUDE ILLNESS PROPHYLAXIS	For all travelers at moderate to high risk for altitude illness including those planning rapid ascents of > 1,600 ft (sleeping altitude) above 9,800ft with/ without extra acclimatization days every 3,300 ft or those with history of altitude illness. • Usual dosing: 125 mg (or 250 mg if >100 kg) twice daily beginning 1 day prior to ascent, during ascent, & for 2 days at destination altitude.

References
1. Centers for Disease Control and Prevention. CDC Health Information for International Travel 2018. New York: Oxford University Press; 2017.
2. Nelson NP, Link-Gelles R, Hofmeister MG, et al. Update: Recommendations of the Advisory Committee on Immunization Practices for Use of Hepatitis A Vaccine for Postexposure Prophylaxis and for Preexposure Prophylaxis for International Travel. MMWR Morb Mortal Wkly Rep 2018;67: 1216–1220

Ideal Body Weight (IBW)

Calculation	Gender/Notes	Calculation
Ideal Body Weight (in kg)	Male	50 + (2.3 x height in inches over 5 feet)
	Female	45.5 + (2.3 x height in inches over 5 feet)
	Boys ≥ 5 feet tall	39 + (2.27 x height in inches over 5 feet)
	Girls ≥ 5 feet tall	42.2 + (2.27 x height in inches over 5 feet)
	Boys & Girls < 5 feet tall	(Height^2 x 1.65)/1000

Body Mass Index (BMI)

Calculation	Gender/Notes	Calculation
Body Surface Area (BSA) (in m^2)	All	• Mosteller: $\sqrt{([\text{height (cm)} \times \text{weight (kg)}]/3600)}$ • Lam: $\sqrt{([\text{height (in)} \times \text{weight (lb)}]/3131)}$ • DuBois & DuBois: 0.007184 x height (cm)$^{0.725}$ x weight (kg)$^{0.425}$
Body Mass Index (in kg/m^2)	All/metric	• Weight (kg)/[height (m)]^2
	All/imperial	• Weight (lb) x 703/height squared in (in^2)

References

1. Mosteller RD. Simplified calculation of body-surface area [letter]. N Engl J Med. *1987;317(17):1098.*

2. Lam TK, Leung DT. More on simplified calculation of body surface area [letter]. N Engl J Med. *1988;318(17):1130.*

3. DuBois D, DuBois EF. A formula to estimate the approximate surface area if height and weight be known. Arch Int Med. *1916;17:863–71.*

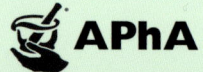

Creatinine Clearance Calculations

Name of Calculation	Formula	Appropriate Use
Cockcroft-Gault	**Women:** $= \dfrac{[(140 - \text{age}) \times \text{weight (in kilograms [kg])}]}{72 \times [\text{serum creatinine in mg/dL}]} \times 0.85$ **Men:** $= \dfrac{[(140 - \text{age}) \times \text{weight (in kilograms [kg])}]}{72 \times [\text{serum creatinine in mg/dL}]}$	• General use in dosing • *Note:* which weight to use in the calculation is based upon the specific drug (ideal, adjusted, or actual body weight) ○ This may require calling the company & may not be in package information. • While serum creatinine may be underestimated in frail or elderly patients, it may be overestimated in muscular patients.
Schwartz	$= \dfrac{[\text{length (in cm)} \times k]}{\text{serum creatinine in mg/dL}}$ <table><tr><td>**Age/Classification**</td><td>**k value to use**</td></tr><tr><td>1 to 52 weeks old</td><td>0.45</td></tr><tr><td>1 to 13 years old</td><td>0.55</td></tr><tr><td>**Females:** 13 to 18 years old</td><td>0.55</td></tr><tr><td>**Males:** 13 to 18 years old</td><td>0.7</td></tr></table>	• Used frequently in pediatric patients • Presents results as mL/minute/1.73m^2
MDRD (Modified Diet in Renal Disease)	Glomerular Filtration Rate: $= 175 \times \text{SCr}^{-1.154} \times \text{age}^{-0.203}$ $\times 1.212$ (if patient is black) $\times 0.742$ (if patient is female)	Used frequently in the staging of patients Not used for acute renal failure While serum creatinine may be underestimated in frail or elderly patients, it may be overestimated in muscular patients.

Recommended Resources/References
1. Cockcroft DW, Gault MH. Prediction of creatinine clearance from serum creatinine. Nephron, 1976. 16(1): 31–41.
2. Schwartz GJ, Haycock GB, Edelmann CM, Spitzer A. A simple estimate of glomerular filtration rate in children derived from body length and plasma creatinine. Pediatrics, 1976. 58:259–263.
3. Levey AS, Stevens LA, Schmid CH, Zhang YL et al. A new equation to estimate glomerular filtration rate. Ann Intern Med, 2009. 150(9): 604–12.

Prepared by Jessica Ramich

69   Peripheral Brain for the Pharmacist

Conversions

Pounds to Kilograms

lb	=	kg	lb	=	kg	lb	=	kg
1	=	0.45	70	=	31.75	140	=	63.50
5		2.27	75		34.02	145		65.77
10		4.54	80		36.29	150		68.04
15		6.80	85		38.56	155		70.31
20		9.07	90		40.82	160		72.58
25		11.34	95		43.09	165		74.84
30		13.61	100		45.36	170		77.11
35		15.88	105		47.63	175		79.38
40		18.14	110		49.90	180		81.65
45		20.41	115		52.16	185		83.92
50		22.68	120		54.43	190		86.18
55		24.95	125		56.70	195		88.45
60		27.22	130		58.91	200		90.72
65		29.48	135		61.24			

Temperature

Fahrenheit to Centigrade or Celsius: $(°F - 32) \times 5/9 = °C$
Centigrade or Celsius to Fahrenheit: $(°C \times 9/5) + 32 = °F$

°C	=	°F	°C	=	°F	°C	=	°F
100.0	=	212.0	39.0	=	102.2	36.8	=	98.2
50.0		122.0	38.8		101.8	36.6		97.9
41.0		105.8	38.6		101.5	36.4		97.5
40.8		105.4	38.4		101.1	36.2		97.2
40.6		105.1	38.2		100.8	36.0		96.8
40.4		104.7	38.0		100.4	35.8		96.4
40.2		104.4	37.8		100.1	35.6		96.1
40.0		104.0	37.6		99.7	35.4		95.7
39.8		103.6	37.4		99.3	35.2		95.4
39.6		103.3	37.2		99.0	35.5		95.0
39.4		102.9	37.0		98.6	0		32.0
39.2		102.6						

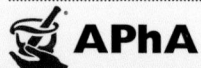

APhA

Weights and Measures

Category	Unit	Conversion
Exact Equivalents	1 ounce (oz)	28.35 grams (g)
	1 pound (lb)	453.6 g (0.4536 kilograms [kg])
	1 fluid oz (fl oz)	29.57 mL
	1 pint (pt)	473.2 mL
	1 quart (qt)	946.4 mL
Metric Conversions	1 kg	1000 g
	1 g	1000 mg
	1 mg	1000 µg
Approximate Measures: Liquids	1 fl oz	30 mL
	1 cup (8 fl oz)	240 mL
	1 pint (16 fl oz)	480 mL
	1 quart (32 fl oz)	960 mL
	1 gallon (128 fl oz)	3800 mL
Approximate Measures: Weights	1 oz	30 g
	1 lb (16 oz)	480 g
	15 grains	1 g
	1 grain	60 mg

Apothecary Equivalents

Category	Unit	Conversion
Weight	1 scruple	20 grains
	60 grains	1 dram
	8 drams	1 ounce
	1 ounce	480 grains
	16 ounces	1 pound (lb)
	1 g	15.43 grains (gr)
	1 gr	64.8 mg
	1 mg	1/65 gr
	0.8 mg	1/80 gr
	0.6 mg	1/100 gr
	0.5 mg	1/120 gr
	0.4 mg	1/150 gr
	0.3 mg	1/200 gr
	0.2 mg	1/300 gr
	0.12 mg	1/500 gr
	0.1 mg	1/600 gr
Volume	60 minims	1 fluidram
	8 fluidrams	1 fluid ounce
	1 fluid once	480 minims
	16 fluid ounces	1 pint (pt)
	1 mL	16.23 minims
	1 minim	0.06 mL

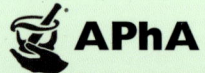

Opioid Conversions

Equianalgesic Dosing

Opioid Agonist	Oral Dose (PO)	Parenteral Dose (IV, SC, IM)	Duration of action (h)
Morphine (IR)	30 mg	10 mg	3 to 4
HYDROmorphone	7.5 mg	1.5 mg	3 to 4
OXYcodone	20 mg	---	3 to 5
HYDROcodone	30 mg	---	3 to 5
OXYmorphone	10 mg	1 mg	3 to 6
Codeine	200 mg	100 mg	4
Fentanyl	---	0.1 mg	2

Note: In use of this table, please consider the following limitations:
1. *Limitation to studies that established equianalgesic dosing: Dosing based upon studies using opioid doses in acute, short-term use. Chronic use requirements may differ for patients. Mean values were often with large variability in potency in study participants. Studies also were based on single dose studies.*
2. *Switching doses may require reducing the dosage of the new agent by 50% (% may vary). Titrate doses to avoid incidence of side effects, particularly with high doses. Monitor patients closely.*
3. *This chart should be used as a guide only. Consider patient-specific factors, such as age, body surface area, organ dysfunction, drug tolerance, type of pain (neuropathic or nociceptive), pharmacogenetics, drug–drug interactions, and drug–food interactions when selecting dosing for patients.*
4. *Conversion risks may exist for patients particularly (e.g., buprenorphine; methadone).*
5. *Some dosing equivalencies may not be bidirectional.*
IR = immediate release.

Reference:
https://rsds.org/wp-content/uploads/2014/12/MEDD-White-Paper-FINAL.pdf
https://www.jpsmjournal.com/article/S0885-3924(09)00630-7/fulltext

Guidance for Changing Opioid Therapy

Step	Description
1	Determine the total 24-hour dose of the currently prescribed analgesic.
2	Convert the currently prescribed opioid to an equivalent dose of the same route (oral vs. parenteral).
3	If pain is controlled, start at 50% to 75% of the equianalgesic dose to account for incomplete cross-tolerance between opioids. If pain is uncontrolled, then start at 100% of the dose.
4	Determine the strength per dose by dividing the dose calculated in Step 4 by the dosing interval. • Choose a dosing interval consistent with the medication duration of action.
5	Provide an appropriate "rescue" dose for breakthrough pain when applicable. • 10% of the total opioid dose given every 1 to 2 hours as needed. • Elderly: rescue dose = 5% of the total opioid dose administered every 4 hours as needed.
6	Titrate baseline and as-needed dose to provide effective pain relief.
7	Use cathartic and stool-softening medications as constipation prophylaxis.

Monitoring for Respiratory Depression
• Unintended increased sedation from opioids is a sign that the patient may be at risk for respiratory depression.

Signs of Respiratory Depression
• Respiratory rate < 10 breaths per minute
• Paradoxic rhythm with little chest expansion
• Evidence of advancing sedation
• Poor respiratory effort or quality
• Snoring or noisy respirations
• Desaturation

Prepared by Jessica Ramich

Systemic Corticosteroid Conversions

Glucocorticoid	Approximate Equivalency	Potency Relative to Hydrocortisone		Half-life T½ (Duration of Action in Hours)	Dosage Forms
		Anti-inflammatory	Mineral Corticoid		
Short Acting					
Cortisone	25 mg	0.8 mg	0.8 mg	8 to 12	PO, IM
Hydrocortisone	20 mg	1 mg	1 mg		IV, IM, PO
Intermediate Acting					
Methylprednisolone	4 mg	5 mg	0.5 mg	12 to 36	IV, IM, PO
Prednisolone	5 mg	4 mg	0.8 mg		IV, PO
Prednisone	5 mg	4 mg	0.8 mg		PO **ONLY**
Triamcinolone	4 mg	5 mg	0 mg		IM, PO
Long Acting					
Betamethasone	0.6 to 0.75 mg	20 to 30 mg	0	36 to 54	IM, PO
Dexamethasone	0.75 mg	20 to 30 mg	0	36 to 72	IV, IM, PO

Note: PO = oral; IM = intramuscular; IV = intravenous.

Suggested References
- *Lexi-Drugs: Corticosteroids Systemic Equivalencies, Drug Monographs*
- *Facts & Comparisons: Equivalencies, Potencies, & T½, Monographs*
- *Micromedex: Drug Monographs*
- *Asare K. Diagnosis & treatment of adrenal insufficiency in the critically ill patient. Pharmacotherapy. 2007 Nov;27(11): 1512–28.*
- *Liu D, Ahmet A, Ward L, et al. A practical guide to the monitoring & management of the complications of systemic corticosteroid therapy. Allergy, Asthma, and Clinical Immunology. 2013. 1, 30.*

Prepared by Jenna Blunt and Jeanine P. Abrons

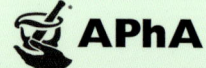

Target Serum Concentrations for Selected Drugs

Reported ranges vary according to source. Ranges reported here are for reference purposes only. Decisions regarding treatment or management of patients should be based on reference intervals reported by the specific laboratory that performs the test. Target ranges represent those for an adult population.

Drug	Target Range
Carbamazepine	4–12 µg/mL
Chloramphenicol	10–20 µg/mL (peak) 5–10 µg/mL (trough) *Note: Levels represent targets for other infections; different targets exist for meningitis*
Cyclosporine	100–400 µg/mL (blood)
Digoxin	Heart Failure–Therapeutic: 0.5–0.8 ng/mL Toxic: levels > 2ng/mL *Note: Levels should be drawn at least 6 to 8 hours after last dose, regardless of route of administration. Specific criteria exist on when to obtain concentration if loading dose is or is not given.*
Ethosuximide	40–100 µg/mL[a]
Lidocaine	Therapeutic: 1.5–5 µg/mL Toxic: > 6 µg/mL
Lithium	Therapeutic: 0.6–1.2 mEq/L Toxic: > 1.5 mEq/L *Note: Different targets exist for acute mania; prevention of episodes in patients with bipolar disorder & elderly patients.*
Phenobarbital	Infants/Children–Therapeutic: 10–40 mcg/mL Adults—Therapeutic: 10–40 µg/mL Toxic: > 40 µg/mL
Phenytoin	10–20 µg/mL[a]
Primidone	5–12 µg/mL[a]
Procainamide/ N-acetylprocainamide (NAPA)	Therapeutic: Procainamide: 4–10 mcg/mL; NAPA: 15–25 mcg/mL Combined: 10–30 mcg/mL
Quinidine	2–5 µg/mL[a]
Theophylline	10–20 µg/mL[a]
Valproic acid	50–100 µg/mL

a. Trough levels just prior to next dose.

Peripheral Brain for the Pharmacist

Normal Laboratory Values[a]

Chemistries

Sodium 135–146 mEq/L	Chloride 95–108 mEq/L	Blood urea nitrogen (BUN) 7–30 mg/dL	Glucose (fasting) ≤ 100 mg/dL
Potassium 3.5–5.3 mEq/L	Bicarbonate 22–29 mEq/L	Creatinine 0.5–1.5 mg/dL	

Hematology

White blood cells
3.8–10.8 × 103/µL

Hemoglobin
13.8–17.2 g/dL (men)
12.0–15.6 g/dL (women)

Hematocrit
41%–50% (men)
35%–46% (women)

Platelets
130–400 × 10³/µL

Test	Component	Normal Range
White Blood Cell (WBC) Differential	Bands	3–5%
	Basophils	0–1%
	Eosinophils	1–3%
	Lymphocytes	23–33%
	Monocytes	3–7%
	Neutrophils	57–67%
	Segmented neutrophils (segs)	54–62%
Red Blood Cell Count	Red blood cell count (men)	$4.4–5.8 \times 10^6/\mu L$
	Red blood cell count (women)	$3.9–5.2 \times 10^6/\mu L$
MCV	Mean corpuscular volume (MCV)	78–102 fL
MCH	Mean corpuscular hemoglobin (MCH)	27–33 pg/cell
MCHC	Mean corpuscular hemoglobin concentration (MCHC)	33–36%
Reticulocytes	Reticulocytes	0.5–2.3%
Arterial Blood Gases	Base excess	±2 mEq/L
	Bicarbonate (HCO_3)	22–26 mEq/L
	Oxygen saturation	94–100%
	Partial pressure of carbon dioxide ($PaCO_2$)	35–45 mmHg
	Partial pressure of oxygen (PaO_2)	75–100 mmHg
	pH	7.35–7.45

Normal Laboratory Values[a] *(continued)*

Test	Component	Normal Range
Comprehensive Metabolic Panel *See Chemistries figure for additional components*	Albumin	3.5–5 g/dL
	Alkaline phosphatase (ALP)	20–125 U/L
	Bilirubin (Total)	≤ 1.3 mg/dL
	Bilirubin (Direct)	≤ 0.4 mg/dL
	Calcium (Total)	8.5–10.3 mg/dL
	Calcium (Ionized)	4.65–5.28 mg/dL
	Carbon dioxide	20–32 mEq/L
	Total serum protein	6.0–8.5 g/dL
Renal Function Panel*	Phosphorus	2.5–4.5 mg/dL
Uric Acid	Uric acid (men)	4.0–8.5 mg/dL
Enzymes	Alanine aminotransferase (ALT)	≤ 48 U/L
	Amylase	30–170 U/L
	Aspartate aminotransferase (AST)	≤ 42 U/L
	Creatine kinase (CK) (men)	≤ 235 U/L
	Creatine kinase (women)	≤ 190 U/L
	Gamma glutamyltransferase (GGT) (men)	≤ 65 U/L
	GGT (women)	≤ 45 U/L
	Lactic acid dehydrogenase (LD or LDH)	≤ 270 U/L
	Lipase	7–60 u/L

a. Values given are for adults. Note that normal laboratory values vary widely between hospitals and laboratories; be sure to check the normal values at your site or institution.
* See also glucose; BUN; BUN/creatinine ratio; calcium; sodium; potassium; chloride; CO_2; albumin

Fluid Composition and Calculations

Patient Monitoring Calculations

Monitoring Component	Values/Description		
Serum Osmolality	mOsm/L = (2 x [Na$^+$]) + ([glucose in mg/dL]/18) + (BUN/2.8)		
Anion Gap (AGE)	Na$^+$ − (Cl$^-$ + HCO$_3^-$)		
Water Deficit	0.6 x body weight (kg) x [1 − (140/Na$^+$)]		
Free Water Deficit (FWD)	Normal total body weight (TBW) − Current TBW		
	Normal TBW (Males) =	Lean body weight (kg) x 0.6 L/kg	
	Normal TBW (Females) =	Lean body weight (kg) x 0.5 L/kg	
	Current TBW =	Normal TBW (140/Current [Na$^+$])	
Corrected Sodium	Na$^+_{measured}$ + [((Serum glucose − 100)/100) x 1.6]		
Corrected Calcium (based on albumin level)	[(normal albumin − patient's albumin) x 0.8] + patient's measured total Ca^{2+}		
Chloride Deficit	0.4 x weight (kg) x (100 − Cl$^-_{measured}$)		
Bicarbonate Deficit	(0.5 x kg) x (24 − HCO$_{3measured}^-$)		

Note: BUN = blood urea nitrogen.

Composition of Intravenous Fluids Used for Volume Resuscitation

Fluid Type/Fluid Component	Sodium [Na$^+$] in mEq/L	Chloride (Cl$^-$) in mEq/L	mOsm/L	Other
Normal Saline (0.9% NS)	154	154	308	Isotonic
5% Dextrose/0.9% NS	154	154	560	Glucose: 50 g/L
Lactated Ringers (LR)	130	109	273	Potassium: K$^+$ Calcium (Ca^{2+}) Lactate[1]
Dextrose 5% (5% D)	0	0	253	Glucose: 50 g/L
0.45% Normal Saline (1/2 NS)	77	77	154	
Dextrose 5%/0.45% NS	77	77	406	Glucose: 50 g/L

[1] K$^+$: 4mEq/L; Ca^{2+}: 1.5 mEq/L; Lactate: 28 mEq/L; Modified based on information from Merck Manual—Emergency Medicine and Critical Care –Fluid Therapy.

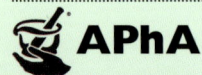
APhA

Electrolytes and Minerals

Laboratory Parameter	Normal Value
Sodium (Na⁺)	135 to 145 mEq/L
Potassium (K⁺)	3.5 to 5 mEq/L
Calcium (Ca²⁺)	8.5 to 10.5 mg/dL
Magnesium (Mg)	1.5 to 2.9 mEq/L
Phosphorus	3.7 to 4.5 mg/dL
Chloride (Cl⁻)	95 to 107 mEq/L
Bicarbonate (HCO₃⁻)	22 to 28 mEq/L
Carbon Dioxide (CO₂)	24 to 32
Blood Urea Nitrogen (BUN)	10 to 20
Serum Creatinine (SCr)	0.5 to 1 mg/dL
Glucose	65 to 99 mg/dL
White Blood Cells (WBC)	3.7 to 10.5 x 10³/µL
Hemoglobin (Hgb)	11.9 to 15.5 g/dL
Hematocrit (Hct)	35 to 47%
Platelets	150 to 400 x 10³/µL
Partial Thrombin Time (PTT)	23 to 31 seconds
Prothrombin Time (PT)	9 to 12 seconds
International Normalized Ratio (INR)	0.9 to 1.1

Note: ranges may vary based on institution-specific laboratory parameters.

Psychiatry Guidelines

Topic Area/ Associated Guideline	Publication/Website	Notes
Major Depressive Disorder	American Psychiatric Association (APA). Practice guideline for the treatment of patients with major depressive disorder. 3rd ed. Arlington (VA): American Psychiatric Association (APA); 2010; http://psychiatryonline.org/pb/assets/raw/sitewide/practiceguidelines/guidelines/mdd.pdf	Updated in 2010
Obsessive-Compulsive Disorder	American Psychiatric Association (APA). Practice guideline for the treatment of patients with obsessive-compulsive disorder. Arlington (VA): American Psychiatric Association (APA); 2007; http://psychiatryonline.org/pb/assets/raw/sitewide/practice_guidelines/guidelines/ocd.pdf	Updated in 2007 (Guideline watch in 2013)
Generalized Anxiety Disorders	National Collaborating Centre for Mental Health, National Collaborating Centre for Primary Care. Generalised anxiety disorder and panic disorder (with or without agoraphobia) in adults. Management in primary, secondary and community care. London (UK): National Institute for Health and Clinical Excellence (NICE); 2011 Jan. 56 p. (Clinical guideline; no. 11) https://www.nice.org.uk/guidance/cg113	Updated in 2011
Panic Disorder	APA. Practice guideline for the treatment of patients with panic disorder. 2nd ed. 2009; http://psychiatryonline.org/pb/assets/raw/sitewide/practice_guidelines/guidelines/panicdisorder.pdf	Updated in 2009
Schizophrenia	APA Practice guideline for the treatment of patients with schizophrenia 2nd ed. http://psychiatryonline.org/pb/assets/raw/sitewide/practice_guidelines/guidelines/schizophrenia.pdf	Updated in 2004 (Guideline watch in 2009)
Bipolar Disorder	APA Practice guideline for the treatment of patients with bipolar disorder. http://psychiatryonline.org/pb/assets/raw/sitewide/practice_guidelines/guidelines/bipolar.pdf	Updated in 2002 (Guideline watch 2005)

Resources for the Practicing Pharmacist

Resource	Website	Use for Pharmacy
Stahl's Essential Psychopharmacology Online	https://stahlonline.cambridge.org	Index available by drug; covers the therapeutic use and mechanisms; guidance on how to select agents; drug interactions; dosing tips; teacher images for presentation
Neuroscience Education Institute	http://neiglobal.com	Information regarding mental health pathophysiology and psychopharmacology; medication comparisons; clinical practice resources
College of Psychiatric and Neurologic Pharmacists	http://cpnp.org	Psychiatric-related job postings; residency information; board certification information; continuing education resources; suggested readings
American Psychiatric Association	http://www.psychiatry.org	Fact brochures; several psychiatry related publications; continuing education resources; clinical practice resources

Prepared by Sara E. Dugan; updates with Jeanine P. Abrons

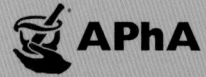

Psychiatric Medications

Medication Class	Common Adverse Drug Reactions	Clinical Pearls
Selective Serotonin Reuptake Inhibitors (SSRIs)	Somnolence; fatigue; insomnia; nausea; dry mouth; diaphoresis; sexual dysfunction; weakness (Fluoxetine); headache	Commonly utilized for the treatment of depression or anxiety disorders. Symptom improvement often takes weeks of therapy. Drug interactions due to CYP inhibition occur with some medications in this class.
Serotonin-Norepinephrine Reuptake Inhibitors (SNRIs)	Fatigue; headache; nausea; dizziness; dry mouth; insomnia; decreased appetite; hyperhidrosis (Desvenlafaxine)	Commonly utilized for the treatment of depression or anxiety disorders. Symptom improvement often takes weeks of therapy. Elevated blood pressure has been reported with some medications in this class.
Tricyclic Antidepressants (TCAs)	Weight gain; sexual dysfunction; hypotension; QT abnormalities; dry mouth; constipation; nausea; somnolence	Commonly utilized for many conditions including depression and anxiety disorders. Symptom improvement often takes weeks of therapy. Tolerability and potential toxicity are a greater concern with this class of medications.
Benzodiazepines	Sedation; dizziness; drowsiness; unsteadiness; hypotension; weakness	Commonly utilized for the treatment of agitation, anxiety, insomnia, or seizure disorders. Improvement is seen relatively quickly. These medications have the potential to cause dependence. Abrupt discontinuation may result in withdrawal seizures.
Second Generation Antipsychotics (SGA)	Sedation; dizziness; hypotension; weight gain; abnormal muscle movements; elevations in glucose or cholesterol levels	Commonly utilized for the treatment of schizophrenia and bipolar disorder, may also be used as adjunct treatment of depression. Monitoring for movement disorders is important to screen for and prevent the development of tardive dyskinesia. Regular metabolic monitoring of blood pressure, weight, glucose, and cholesterol levels is recommended.

Note: CYP = cyctochrome P450.

Prepared by Sara E. Dugan

Nutrition

Harris–Benedict Equation for Basic Metabolic Rate	Ideal Body Weight Equation
Male • 66.47 + (13.7 x kg) + (5 x cm) − (6.7 x years) = kcal/day **Female** • 655.1 + (9.56 x kg) + (1.85 x cm) − (4.68 x years) = kcal/day **Notes** • ↑ metabolic requirements can be factored in by multiplying the kcal/day by an injury factor (between 1 & 2.5)	**Male** • 50 kg + (2.3 kg x inch over 5 ft) **Female** • 45.5 kg + (2.3 kg x inch over 5 ft)

Enteral Nutrition	
Indications for Use "If the gut works, use it."	• Failed swallow evaluation • Esophageal mass • Intubation • Unable to meet oral (PO) intake needs • Functioning gastrointestinal (GI) tract
Sample Indications for Frequency (Duration) *Select option best for patient care*	**Continuous (24 hours)** • With initiation of enteral feeds • With labile blood sugars difficult to manage on cyclic/bolus feeds **Nocturnal or cyclic (12 to 16 hours)** • If tube feeds (TF) are used to supplement oral intake. • If TF tolerated at a higher rate: will allow more time away from feeding pump **Bolus (never an option with J-tubes)** • To simulate routine meal time schedule

Total Parenteral Nutrition (TPN)	
Indications for Use	• Nonfunctioning GI tract • Necessity for bowel rest • GI obstruction • GI dysfunction/malabsorption • Significant GI resection
Calculating TPN	• Weight based • Access-site dependent (central vs. peripheral) 1. Determine macronutrients 2. Determine electrolytes (based on daily labs & predicted daily requirements) 3. Determine volume/fluid needs
Ordering TPN	• Reassess electrolytes & blood sugars daily • Monitor kidney function, volume status, & current patient presentation
Weaning TPN	• ↓ rate by 50% every 20 minutes over 1 hour • Continue TPN until > 60% of PO diet is tolerated • Obtain blood glucose 1 hour after TPN is discontinued

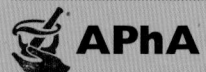
APhA

Nutrition *(continued)*

Component	Standard Requirement	Commonly Formulated within Parenteral Nutrition Solutions
Common Daily Requirements for Parenteral Nutrition		
Water	25 to 40 mL/kg	
Calcium	10 to 15 mEq	Calcium gluconate; calcium chloride
Magnesium	8 to 20 mEq	Magnesium sulfate; magnesium chloride
Phosphorus	20 to 40 mmol	Sodium phosphate; potassium phosphate
Potassium	1 to 2 mEq/kg	Potassium chloride; potassium acetate; potassium phosphate
Sodium	1 to 2 mEq/kg	Sodium chloride; sodium acetate; sodium phosphate
Acetate	As needed to maintain acid-base balance	Sodium acetate; potassium acetate
Chloride	As needed to maintain acid-base balance	Sodium chloride; potassium chloride; magnesium chloride; calcium chloride

Reference: Mirtallo J, Canada T, Johnson D, et al. Safe Practices for Parenteral Nutrition. Journal of Parenteral and Enteral Nutrition, 6, S39-70. 2004.

Consideration	Information
Miscellaneous Monitoring Associated with Total Parenteral Nutrition (TPN)	
Albumin	3 weeks half life
Prealbumin	2 day half life
Complete metabolic panel (CMP) Complete blood counts (CBC)	Monitor daily during acute inpatient hospitalization. As patient stabilizes or goes home on TPN, labs can be done less frequently (twice weekly, weekly, or bi-weekly).
Lipid panel	Monitored frequently during acute inpatient hospitalization in patients receiving lipid emulsion therapy
Vitamins, minerals	Check if a deficiency is suspected; otherwise consider yearly
Central line infection	Patients should be educated on signs/symptoms of an infection in their central line so they can conduct daily surveillance (redness, tenderness, oozing, fever, chills, swelling, pain). If an infection is suspected, it is important that the patient seek medical attention in a timely fashion.

Sample References
1. Kreymann KG, Berger MM, Deutz NE, et al. ESPEN Guidelines on Enteral Nutrition: Intensive Care. Clin Nutrition, 2006. 25(2):210–23.
2. Madsen H, Frankel EH. The Hitchhiker's Guide to Parenteral Nutrition Management for Adult Patients. Practical Gastroenterology, 2006. 46–68.
3. Barnadas G. Navigating Home Care: Parenteral Nutrition – Part 2. Practical Gastroenterology, 2003. https://med.virginia.edu/ginutrition/wp-content/uploads/sites/199/2015/11/practicalgastro-nov03.pdf (accessed November 2018).

Nutrition *(continued)*

Calculating TPN	
Step	**Description of Step**
1. Calculate Energy (Caloric) Needs	• Use the Harris-Benedict equation + activity + stress factor = energy (kcal) or you may use a scale. ○ The calories from protein, carbohydrates, and lipids should add up to this total.

Patient Description *Notes*	Energy Needs (Caloric) *Note: use actual body weight unless otherwise specified*
Well nourished, healthy, & requires maintenance therapy	• 20 to 25 kcal/kg
Critically ill; has metabolic stress; with recent trauma or is undernourished	• 25 to 30 kcal/kg

Critically ill & obese (BMI ≥ 30)
• *Consider permissive underfeeding, hypocaloric high-protein feeding, or eucaloric feeding*
	• Using actual body weight:
	  11 to 14 kcal/kg
	OR
	• Using ideal body weight:
	  22 to 25 kcal/kg

Acute renal failure or chronic kidney disease (CKD)	• 25 to 30 kcal/kg

Calculating TPN	
2. Determine Protein Needs	• High protein content may be more appropriate during the acute stages of critical illness • To calculate grams (g) of protein supplied in a solution, multiply total volume of amino acids (in mL) by the amino acid concentration. • Protein provides ~ 4 kcal/gram.

Patient Description *Notes*	Protein Requirements *Note: Use ideal body weight*
Well nourished, healthy, & requires maintenance therapy	• 0.8 to 1 g/kg
Critically ill; has metabolic stress; with recent trauma or is undernourished	• 1.2 to 2 g/kg
Critically ill & obese (BMI ≥ 30) • *Consider permissive underfeeding, hypocaloric high-protein feeding or eucaloric feeding*	• BMI of 30 to 40: 2 g/kg • BMI > 40: 2.5 g/kg
Acute renal failure or chronic kidney disease (CKD)	• Acute kidney injury (AKI) + intermittent hemodialysis (iHD): 1.2 to 2 g/kg • CRRT: 2 to 2.5 g/kg • CKD Stage 3 or 4, not acutely ill: 0.3 to 0.6 g/kg • CKD Stage 5 with iHD 3 times per week: 1.2 g/kg • CKD Stage 5 with peritoneal dialysis daily: 1.3 g/kg

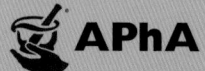
APhA

Nutrition *(continued)*

Step	Description of Step
3. Calculate the Fat (Lipids) Needed Based on Total Energy Needs	• Fat needs: 1 to 2.5 g of fat/kg or 15–30% of nonprotein kcal (maximum tolerance of 2.5 g/kg body weight & 60% of energy from fat) • Fat: 9 kcal/gram • Common caloric intake of available formulation: {{TABLE}}
4. Calculate the Carbohydrates (CHO)	• Determine needs by subtracting fat (lipid) needs & protein calorie needs from total energy (caloric) needs. Remaining amount is needed kcal from CHO. Take kcal CHO needed/kcal per 1 L of dextrose solution = mL dextrose solution needed. • Dextrose monohydrate = 3.4 kcal/g • Determine energy content of 1 L of formulate by multiplying mL x percentage of dextrose in dextrose solution. ○ Common formulations: dextrose 50% 1 L = 1,700 kcal; dextrose 70% 1 L = 2,380 kcal • Maximum rate of administration should not exceed 5 mg CHO/kg/min (could lead to hyperglycemia, liver dysfunction, and increase CO_2 production)
5. Calculate the Fluid Needs	• Fluid-restricted formulas with higher caloric density (kcal/mL) are available but may cause ↑ diarrhea due to ↑ osmolality • Fluid needs: 25–35 mL/kg/day x feeding weight (kg) = fluid needs/day (mL)
6. Determine Electrolyte Needs	Consider determining electrolyte formulations in the following order: (1) phosphate (sodium or potassium), (2) potassium (acetate or chloride), (3) sodium (acetate or chloride), (4) magnesium, and (5) calcium in order to take formulations into consideration efficiently

7. Determine Vitamin, Mineral, & Additives	• Vitamin solutions include 12 vitamins.
	• Trace elements include copper, zinc, manganese, chromium, and selenium.
	  ○ Cholestasis: caution with manganese and copper—consider dose reduction or omission
	  ○ Renal dysfunction: caution with chromium use—consider reduction or omission
	• Other additives may include insulin, H2 receptor antagonists, and iron as examples.

Table inside Step 3:

Lipid Formulation	10% fat emulsion	20% fat emulsion	30% fat emulsion
Kcal/mL	1.1 kcal/mL	2 kcal/mL	3 kcal/mL

Peripheral Brain for the Pharmacist

Nutrition *(continued)*

Factors to Consider When Calculating TPN	
Factor	**Consideration**
Macronutrient Complexity	• Consider patient's ability to break down, absorb, & tolerate macronutrients
Disease Specific	• Consider whether the product is designed for a specific disease state
Obesity	• ASPEN/SCCM guidelines recommend obese patients (body mass index [BMI] >30 kg/m^2) should receive 11 to 14 kcal/kg (actual weight) or 22 to 25 kcal/kg (ideal weight); protein requirements should be dosed based upon ideal body weight (IBW)
Allergies	• Lipid emulsion products currently made from soybeans/eggs: contraindicated in patients with severe allergies to soybean/egg

Note: ASPEN = American Society for Parenteral and Enteral Nutrition; SCCM = Society of Critical Care Medicine.

Refeeding Syndrome	
Consideration	**Information**
Refeeding Syndrome General Information	• Occurs when carbohydrates are introduced to body → insulin to be released & electrolytes to be driven into cells (→ ↓ serum levels)
Risk Factors	• Body mass index (BMI) <18.5; unintentional weight loss > 10% in 3 months; little/no intake for > 5 days; low electrolyte levels prior to initiation of nutrition therapy
Prevention	• Slow nutrition titration • Close electrolyte monitoring (including K$^+$, Mg^{2+}, and P$^+$) • Patients with refeeding syndrome also experience acute thiamine deficiency due to Krebs cycle; give thiamine to at-risk patients to prevent natural depletion with administration of carbohydrates
Treatment	• Urgent repletion of electrolytes depending on the severity of lab values (including differences in dosing and formulation)

Reference: Mehanna HM, Moledina J, Travis J. Refeeding syndrome: what it is, and how to prevent and treat it. BMJ 2008; 336:1495.

Prepared by Jenna Blunt and Jeanine P. Abrons

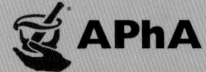

Chronic Kidney Disease

Chronic Kidney Disease (CKD) Staging

Stage	GFR	Description	Management
Stage 1	≥ 90	Kidney damage (with normal or ↑ GFR)	Diagnosis and treatment of comorbid conditions; ↓ progression; cardiovascular risk reduction
Stage 2	60–89	Kidney damage (with mild ↓ GFR)	Estimating progression
Stage 3	30–59	Moderate ↓ GFR	Evaluating and treating complications
Stage 4	15–29	Severe ↓ GFR	Preparation for replacement therapy
Stage 5	< 15 (or dialysis)	Kidney failure	Replacement therapy by dialysis or transplantation (if uremia present)

Note: GFR=glomerular filtration rate in mL/min/1.73m²

Management of Comorbid Conditions with CKD

Condition	Goal	Resource
Diabetes	Hgb_{A1C} ~ 7 %	National Kidney Foundation (NKF). KDOQI Clinical Practice Guideline for Diabetes & CKD: 2012 Update. *Am J Kidney Dis.* 2012 Nov;60(5):850–86.
Hypertension	< 140/90 mmHg	KDIGO Clinical Practice Guideline for the Management of Blood Pressure in CKD. *Kidney Int Suppl.* 2012 Dec;2(5):337–414.
Proteinuria	< 3 mg/mmol	KDIGO Clinical Practice Guideline for the Evaluation and Management of CKD. *Kidney Int Suppl.* 2013 Jan; 3(1):1–150.
Dyslipidemia	LDL < 100 mg/dL TG < 150 mg/dL	KDIGO Clinical Practice Guideline for Lipid Management in CKD. *Kidney Int Suppl.* 2013 Nov;3(3):259–305.
Anemia	Hgb > 11 g/dL	National Clinical Guideline Centre. Anemia Management in People with CKD. London (UK): NICE; 2011 Feb. 38. KDIGO Anemia Work Group. KDIGO Clinical Practice Guideline for Anemia in CKD. *Kidney Int Suppl.* 2012 Aug;2(4):279–335.
Metabolic Bone Disease	Ca^{2+}: 8.4 to 9.5 mg/dL PO^4: • 2.7 to 4.6 mg/dL (Stages 3 & 4) • 3.5 to 5.4 (Stage 5)	NICE. Hyperphosphataemia in CKD. Management of Hyperphosphataemia in Patients with Stage 4 or 5 CKD. London (UK): NICE; 2013 Mar. 22. KDIGO CKD-MBD Work Group. KDIGO Clinical Practice Guideline for the Diagnosis, Evaluation, Prevention, and Treatment of CKD–Mineral and Bone Disorder (MBD). *Kidney Int.* 2009 Aug; 76 (Suppl 113):S1–130.

Note: Hgb = hemoglobin; LDL = low-density lipoprotein; TG = triglycerides; KDIGO = Kidney Disease Improving Global Outcomes; NICE = National Institute for Health & Clinical Excellence.

References
1. National Kidney Foundation Clinical Practice Guidelines for CKD: evaluation, classification and stratification. New York, NY. 2002.
2. Johnson CA, Levey AS, Coresh J, et al. Clinical practice guidelines for chronic kidney disease in adults: Part I. Definition, disease stages, evaluation, treatment, and risk factors. Am Fam Physician. 2004 Sep 1;70(5):869–76.
3. Levey AS, Coresh J, Balk E, et al. National Kidney Foundation practice guidelines for CKD: evaluation, classification, and stratification. Ann Intern Med. 2003 Jul 15;139(2):137–47.
4. Bailie GR, Uhlig K, Levey AS. Clinical practice guidelines in nephrology: evaluation, classification, and stratification of CKD. Pharmacotherapy. 2005 Apr;25(4):491–502.

Prepared by Jessica Ramich

Acute Pain Management

Pain Assessment Tools:
- 0 to 10 numeric rating scale (NRS)
- Wong-Baker FACES® Pain Rating Scale: http://wongbakerfaces.org/ (Accessed 2019)
- Visual analog scale (VAS)
- COMFORT Scale
- CRIES scale (Crying, oxygenation, vital signs, facial expression and sleeplessness) (Pediatric)
- MOBID-2 (Dementia)
- FLACC (Face, Legs, Activity, Cry and Consolability) Score
- Brief Pain Inventory (BPI)

World Health Organization Treatment Ladder

Step 1
Mild to Moderate Pain:
Use nonopioid analgesics (e.g., acetaminophen, nonsteroidal anti-inflammatories) ± adjuvant analgesics

Step 2
Moderate or Persistent Pain Unrelieved by Step 1:
If patient's pain is unrelieved by Step 1: Use low-dose opioid therapy ± nonopioids ± adjuvant analgesics

Step 3
Severe or Persistent Pain Unrelieved by Step 2:
If patient's pain is unrelieved by Step 2: Schedule opioids ± non-opioids ± adjuvant analgesics

Term	Definition	Examples
Non-opioids	Pain medications often used in the treatment of mild to moderate pain that do not have opioid properties.	Acetaminophen; ibuprofen; naproxen; aspirin
Opioids	A type of medication related to opium with analgesic properties.	Morphine, codeine, oxycodone, hydromorphone, buprenorphine, methadone, fentanyl, oxymorphone, hydrocodone, tramadol, tapentadol
Adjuvant- Neuropathic pain	Drugs primarily indicated for other conditions but found to have benefit in pain management.	Antidepressants (e.g., serotonin norepinephrine uptake inhibitors, tricyclic antidepressants); calcium channel alpha 2-delta ligands (e.g., gabapentin, pregabalin); topical therapy (e.g., lidocaine); sodium channel blockers (e.g., carbamazepine, oxcarbazepine)

Common Adverse Effects of Opioids
Constipation, nausea/vomiting, sedation, cognitive impairment, pruritus, dry mouth

Other Possible Adverse Effects of Opioids
Respiratory depression, dependence, allergy, pruritus, seizures, urinary retention, delirium, hyperalgesia

Resources
- Schneider C, Yale SH, Larson M. Principles of Pain Management. *Clin Med Res.* 2003; 1(4): 337–340.
- National Institutes of Health (NIH): Pain Consortium: https://painconsortium.nih.gov/ (Accessed 2019)
- American Academy of Pain Medicine: https://painmed.org/clinician-resource-for-pain-medicine (Accessed 2019)
- JAMA Patient Page: Acute Pain Treatment. *JAMA.* 2008; 299(1): 128.
- Agency Medical Directors Group. Interagency Guideline on Opioid Dosing for Chronic Non-Cancer Pain (CNCP): 2010.
- Equianalgesic Dosing of Opioids for Pain Management. Pharmacist's Letter. August 2012.
- Gippsland Region Palliative Care Consortium Clinical Practice Group. Opioid Conversion Guidelines. February 2011.
- https://www.cdc.gov/drugoverdose/pdf/calculating_total_daily_dose-a.pdf (Acessed 2019)

Dosages at or above 50 morphine milligram equivalents (MME)/day increase risks for overdose by at least 2 times

Prepared by Jessica Ramich; updates by Jeanine Abrons

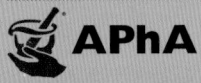

Veterinary Medicine Information

Key Facts
- Dosing usually weight based.
- More than 50% of U.S. households have a companion animal (pets are more common than children).
- Many antibiotics are available to animals as an over-the-counter (OTC) product.
- Must have a valid veterinarian-client-patient relationship.

Veterinary Consideration	Description
Differences Between Common Pets	• Dogs (canines) more commonly have hypothyroidism. • Cats (felines) more commonly have hyperthyroidism.
Counseling	**Insulin Administration Technique** • Inject at a 45° angle under skin around neck of a dog or cat (e.g., where a mom cat carries her kittens). • Keep needle parallel to skin & inject under loose skin between neck & back. • Subcutaneous is preferred; intramuscular (IM) administration is an option (administer IM in thigh) but not preferred due to nerve damage risk. ○ Further details: http://www.peteducation.com (accessed December 2017) **SIG Abbreviations** • Vary for humans & animals (e.g., once daily: humans = QD; animals = SID)
Dosing Considerations	• Pain medications/antibiotics dosed higher & more often (different from humans).

Toxicity	• Ingestion (accidental or overdose) of some OTC products may be toxic to pets.
	   ○ Acetaminophen example: cat (feline) toxic dose = > 10 mg/kg; dog (canine) = > 200 mg/kg
	     ○ Treatment: N-acetylcysteine; cimetidine within 48 hours

Compounding	• FDA Regulations & Compliance Policy Guide 608.400 "Compounding of Drugs for Use in Animals." • For a compounding prescription to be valid for a pet, a valid relationship must exist between provider & patient (pet/owner) • Veterinary medicines may be compounded when no approved animal or human drug is available. • A beyond-use date should be assigned as indicated for the product.

Drug, Dosing, & Pharmacology Resources
- National Animal Poison Control Center: www.aspca.org/pet-care/poison-control
- Plumb's Veterinary Drug Handbook
- American Veterinary Medical Association—Compounding: https://www.avma.org/KB/Policies/Pages/Compounding.aspx
- https://dailymed.nlm.nih.gov/dailymed/

Veterinary Disease States
- Petplace.com
- www.petcoach.com

Legal & Regulatory Resources
- Food & Drug Association (FDA)/Center for Veterinary Medicine (CVM): http://www.fda.gov/AnimalVeterinary

Prepared by Breanna Sunderman

Quality, Free Online Resources

Resource	Features or Benefit	Limitations in Use
U.S. Food and Drug Administration (FDA) http://www.fda.gov/	• Animal Drugs@FDA (Green Book) • Therapeutic Equivalence Evaluations (Orange Book) • Drugs@FDA • FDA Drug Shortages • National Drug Code Directory	The large amount of information may make navigation difficult.
U.S. National Library of Medicine (NLM) https://www.nlm.nih.gov/	• MEDLINE/PubMed/MedlinePlus • ClinicalTrials.gov • DailyMed • Pillbox • Populations & genetics information • Environmental health & toxicology	The connection or overlap of information between libraries; cross-referencing is improving.
Drugs.com https://www.drugs.com	• ~24,000 monographs from Wolters Kluwer Health, American Society of Health-System Pharmacists, Cerner Multum, & Micromedex from Truven Health	This website may appear cluttered. Commercial advertising is accepted.
Medscape: Drugs & Diseases http://reference.medscape.com	• ~ 7,100 monographs based on FDA approvals	Information is abbreviated & may not be comprehensive.
Merck Manuals http://www.merckmanuals.com/	• Drug monographs from Wolters Kluwer Clinical Drug Information, Inc. • Consumer/Professional Version • Veterinary Edition	Publication reflects medical practice & information in the United States. It does not include international perspectives.
Centers for Disease Control and Prevention (CDC) http://www.cdc.gov/	• Morbidity & Mortality Weekly Report • Free travel apps: TravWell; Can I Eat This?; 2018 Yellow Book	Lots of information but easy navigation.
Drug Enforcement Administration (DEA) https://www.dea.gov	• Drugs of Abuse	Focused on enforcement of controlled substances laws & U.S. regulations; not global.
World Health Organization (WHO) http://www.who.int/en/	• International Pharmacopoeia • World Health Report • International Travel & Health • International Classification of Diseases-10	The website's expansive coverage makes navigation difficult.
Institute for Safe Medication Practices (ISMP) http://www.ismp.org	• ISMP Guidelines • Medication Error Reporting • Medication safety tools and resources	The organization provides independent oversight. It relies on donations & grants. Subscriptions are fee based.
Agency for Healthcare Research and Quality (AHRQ) http://www.ahrq.gov/	• Health Literacy Center	Lots of information but easy to navigate.

Note: All sites accessed November 2018.

Prepared by Vern Duba & Jeanine P. Abrons

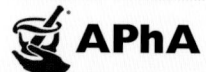

National Clinical Guidelines

Cardiovascular Section Guidelines

Guideline (Publication Date)	Recognized Source of Guideline
Antithrombotic and Thrombolytic Therapy (2016)	American College of Chest Physicians (CHEST)
Blood Cholesterol (2018)	American College of Cardiology and American Heart Association (ACC/AHA)
Heart Failure (2017) **Acute (2014); Chronic (2018)**	American College of Cardiology, American Heart Association, and Heart Failure Society of America (ACC/AHA/HFSA) National Institute for Health and Care Excellence (NICE)
Hypertension (2017)	American College of Cardiology and American Heart Association (ACC/AHA)
Lifestyle Management to Reduce Cardiovascular Risk (2013)	American College of Cardiology and American Heart Association (ACC/AHA)
Myocardial Infarction (MI) (2013, 2014, 2015)	American College of Cardiology and American Heart Association (ACC/AHA)
Overweight and Obesity (2013)	American College of Cardiology, American Heart Association, The Obesity Society (ACC/AHA/TOS)
Stroke (2018) Guidelines also exist for prevention	American Heart Association and American Stroke Association (AHA/ASA)

Endocrine Section Guidelines

Guideline (Publication Date)	Recognized Source of Guideline
Diabetes (2018)—rolling updates	American Diabetes Association (ADA)
Endocrine (multiple years)	American Association of Clinical Endocrinologists and American College of Endocrinology (AACE/ACE)

Respiratory Section Guidelines

Guideline (Publication Date)	Recognized Source of Guideline
Asthma (GINA 2018)	Global Initiative for Asthma (GINA)
Chronic Obstructive Pulmonary Disease (2017)	Global Initiative for Chronic Obstructive Lung Disease (GOLD)

National Clinical Guidelines *(continued)*

Infectious Diseases Section Guidelines

Guideline (Publication Date)	Where to Access
Community-Acquired Pneumonia (CAP) (2007)	Infectious Diseases Society of America
Hospital-Acquired Pneumonia (HAP) (2016)	Infectious Diseases Society of America
Clostridium difficile (2018)	Infectious Diseases Society of America
Other (multiple years)	Infectious Diseases Society of America

Special Populations Section Guidelines

Guideline (Publication Date)	Where to Access
Beers Criteria (2015)	American Geriatrics Society
Pharmacological Management of Persistent Pain in Older Persons (2009)	American Geriatrics Society
Prevention of Falls in Older Persons (2010)	American Geriatrics Society

Miscellaneous Section Guidelines

Guideline (Publication Date)	Where to Access
General	
Mental Health	
Alzheimer's Disease (2011)	https://www.alz.org/health-care-professionals/clinical-guidelines-dementia-care.asp

Prepared by Jeanine P. Abrons

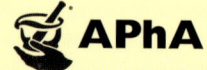

Clinically Significant Drug Interactions

Category/ Classification	Electronic Resource
Cytochrome P450 Drug Interactions	Indiana University Division of Clinical Pharmacology P450 Drug Interaction Table *(http://medicine.iupui.edu/clinpharm/ddis/main-table/)*
QTc-Prolonging Medications	Arizona Center for Education and Research on Therapeutics *(https://www.crediblemeds.org/index.php/login/dlcheck)* Free registration now required
Grapefruit Interactions with Medications	University of Washington *(https://www.washington.edu/research/research-centers/center-of-excellence-for-natural-product-drug-interaction-napdi-research/)* FDA *(http://www.fda.gov/ForConsumers/consumerupdates/ucm292276.htm)*
General Interactions Including Herbals	University of Maryland Drug Interaction Checker *(http://umm.edu/health/medical/drug-interaction-tool)*
Oral Contraception Interactions/ Pregnancy	Reprotox *(http://www.reprotox.org/Default.aspx)* Additional resources listed in "Special Populations" section; Note: paid resource
Herbal Information	National Center for Complementary and Alternative Medicine *(http://nccam.nih.gov/health/herbsataglance.htm)*
Dietary Supplements	National Center for Complementary and Alternative Medicine *(http://nccam.nih.gov/health/supplements/wiseuse.htm)*

All websites accessed November 2018.

Prepared by Jeanine P. Abrons

Medications with Adverse Withdrawal Effects from Abrupt Discontinuation

Medication Category	Medication Examples	Presentation with Abrupt Stop	Symptoms	Management/Risk Factors	Evidence	Potential to be Life Threatening
Anticonvulsant	Gabapentin (Neurontin®) Pregabalin (Lyrica®) Phenytoin (Dilantin®)	Seizures; anxiety; insomnia; nausea; pain; sweating	Mild to Severe	**Management** • Taper over at least 2 to 4 weeks	Good	YES
Anti-Parkinson	Carbidopa/Levodopa (Sinemet®) Amantadine (Symmetrel®) Rasagiline (Azilect®)	Hyperpyrexia; confusion; muscle rigidity; tachycardia; tachypnea	Severe	**Management** • Taper over ~ 4 weeks	Good	YES
Alpha Agonist	Clonidine (Catapres®)	Rebound hypertension; tachycardia; agitation; headache; stroke (rarely); encephalopathy (rarely)	Mild to Severe	**Management** • Taper over 1 to 2 weeks **Risk factors** • Use > 1 month, cardiovascular disease, β-blocker use, daily dose > 1.2 mg	Excellent	YES
Antipsychotic	Clozapine (Clozaril®) Quetiapine (Seroque®) Olanzapine (Zyprexa®) Risperidone (Risperda®) Haloperidol (Haldol®)	Sweating; salivation; flu symptoms; paresthesia; bronchoconstriction; urination; gastrointestinal; anorexia; vertigo; insomnia, agitation/ anxiety; restlessness; movement disorders, psychosis	Mild to Severe	**Management** • No > 50% ↓ every 2 weeks • May stop more abruptly in hospital • If switching agent, may cross-taper: ↓ dose of old agent while titrating up new agent at ~ same rate (e.g. over 2 to 3 weeks)	Excellent	NO
Beta Blocker	Atenolol (Tenormin®) Bisoprolol (Zebeta®) Metoprolol (multiple) Propranolol (Inderal®)	Hypertension; angina; myocardial infarction, ventricular arrhythmia	Mild to Severe	**Management** • ↓ dosage over 1 to 2 weeks & up to 3 weeks with history of myocardial infarction	Good	YES

Updated by Angela Wojtczak, Joanna Rusch, Elisha Andreas, and Jeanine P. Abrons.

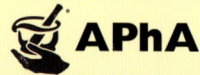

94

Medications with Adverse Withdrawal Effects from Abrupt Discontinuation (continued)

Medication Category	Medication Examples	Presentation with Abrupt Stop	Symptoms	Management/Risk Factors	Evidence	Potential to be Life Threatening
Benzodiazepine and "Z drugs"	Alprazolam (Xanax®) Clonazepam (Klonopin®) Lorazepam (Ativan®) Triazolam (Halcion) Eszopiclone (Lunesta) Zolpidem (Ambien)	Sweating; tremor; agitation; nausea; tachycardia; insomnia; anxiety; vomiting; hallucinations; seizures	Mild to Severe	• **Risk factors** · High-dose, long-term use · Use of short-acting agent • **Management** · Taper or sub long-acting agent over 2 to 3 months	Excellent	YES
Butalbital Combination Products	Fiorinal Fioricet	Headache exacerbation; delirium; tremors; seizures	Mild to Severe	• **Risk factors** · Constant, long-term use of ≥ 7 doses daily • **Management** · Taper over 4 to 6 weeks. With ≥ 12 doses daily, consider referral.	Fair	YES
Corticosteroid	Prednisone (Deltasone®) Methylprednis (Solu-Medrol®) Hydrocortisone (Cortef®)	Adrenal insufficiency—nausea; vomiting; fatigue; weakness; ↓ appetite; ↓ weight; hypoglycemia; ↓ mood; adrenal crisis	Mild to Severe	• **Risk factor** · Prednisone > 7.5 mg daily for > 3 weeks • **Management** · Based on institution; taper over 2 months for pituitary-adrenal response recovery	Excellent	YES
Nitrate	Isosorbide mononitrate & dinitrate (Imdur®, Isordil®)	Rebound angina	Mild to Severe	• **Management** · Consider taper over 1 to 2 weeks, use sublingual nitroglycerine as needed	Fair – Good	NO
Opioid	Oxycodone (OxyContin®) Hydrocodone (Hysingla®) Codeine Morphine (MS Contin®)	Flulike symptoms; insomnia; anxiety; cramps; fatigue; malaise	Mild to Severe	• **Management** · Taper over 2 to 3 weeks if severe adverse effects, overdose, or with abuse · Taper by ≤ 10% of original dose per week	Good	NO

Updated by Angela Wojtczak, Joanna Rusch, Elisha Andreas, and Jeanine P. Abrons.

Medications with Adverse Withdrawal Effects from Abrupt Discontinuation *(continued)*

Medication Category	Medication Examples	Presentation with Abrupt Stop	Symptoms	Management/Risk Factors	Evidence	Potential to be Life Threatening
Nitrate	Isosorbide mononitrate & dinitrate (Imdur®, Isordil®)	Rebound angina	Mild to Severe	• **Management** · Consider taper over 1 to 2 weeks, use sublingual nitroglycerine as needed	Fair – Good	NO
Opioid	Oxycodone (OxyContin®) Hydrocodone (Hysingla®) Morphine (MS Contin®)	Flulike symptoms; insomnia; anxiety; cramps; fatigue; malaise	Mild to Severe	• **Management** · Taper over 2 to 3 weeks if severe adverse effects, overdose, or with abuse · Taper by ≤ 10% of original dose per week	Good	NO
Antidepressant	Duloxetine (Cymbalta®) Paroxetine (Paxil®) Sertraline (Zoloft®) Venlafaxine (Effexor®) Desvenlafaxine (Pristiq®)	Flulike symptoms; insomnia; nausea; imbalance; sensory disturbances; hyper-arousal (FINISH)	Mild to Moderate	• **Risk factors** · > 6 weeks use or short T½ • **Management** · ↓ dose over weeks to months · Sub longer acting agent & ↓ every 2 to 3 weeks. · ↓ based on indication	Good	NO
Carbamate	Carisoprodol (Soma®)	Body aches; sweats; palpitations; anxiety; restlessness; insomnia	Mild to Moderate	• **Management** · Long taper: renal or liver impairment, age > 65, TDD > 1400 mg, taper over 9 days* (specific taper schedule available) · Short taper: taper over 4 days*	Fair	NO

Notes: References available upon request. List may not represent all medications that have negative effects with abrupt discontinuation.

↑ Classification of discontinuation symptoms & documentation based on the following criteria
- *Documentation: Excellent = package inserts, clinical trials, case reports/case series, reported & evaluated frequently in clinical literature; Good = package inserts, clinical trials, case reports/ case series, reported & evaluated minimally in clinical literature; Fair = package inserts, case reports/case series, reported & evaluated minimally in clinical literature.*
- *Discontinuation symptom severity: Severe = potentially life threatening with abrupt stopping; Moderate = bothersome, slightly less severe & non-life threatening symptoms; Mild = less severe symptoms but withdrawal reaction present.*

Updated by Angela Wojtczak, Joanna Rusch, Elisha Andreas, and Jeanine P. Abrons.

APhA

FASTHUG-MAIDENS: Approach to Identifying Drug-Related Problems (DRPs) & Aspects of Critical Care for Intensive Care Units (ICU) Pharmacists

SIDE 1 – FASTHUG

Letter	Area of Care	Role	Examples
F	Feeding	• Discuss feeding route needs. • Medication route changes. • Monitor electrolytes. • Suggest alterations to feeding/supplementation based upon lab results.	• Oral preferred before enteral nutrition before parenteral nutrition • Consider formulation challenges (e.g., crushing medications) • PO (oral) to IV or IV to PO conversions
A	Analgesia	• Assess pain using a pain scale. • Adequate analgesic but not excessive. • Avoid excessive analgesia to minimize respiratory depression. • Opioids + bowel regimen.	• Pain scales: Wong-Baker FACES/Visual Analog Scale/Brief Pain Inventory • Monitor other ways to assess pain in ICU: grimacing; ↑BP, tachycardia • Side effects to consider: Respiratory depression, constipation, hypotension, hallucinations & rash
S	Sedation	• Initiate, discontinue, adjust doses of sedative medications. • Assess sedation as a continuous infusion, intermittent dosing, & as needed. • Avoid excessive sedation to minimize risk of venous thrombosis, intestinal dysmotility	• MV is uncomfortable. • Monitor for: Propofol Infusion Syndrome (PRIS) = cardiac/renal failure & rhabdomyolysis, & hypertriglyceridemia • Short-term sedation: propofol vs. Long-term sedation: midazolam, lorazepam
T	Thromboembolic prophylaxis	• Initiate to almost all patients, unless presence of intracranial or active gastrointestinal bleeding	• LMWH, UFH, compression devices, intravascular filters
H*	Head of bed elevation; Hyperdelirium & Hypodelirium	• Minimize risk of aspiration pneumonia. • Assess using tools such as Intensive Care Delirium Screening Checklist or Confusion Assessment Method for the ICU.	• Head of bed inclined at 45° to ↓ gastroesophageal reflex in mechanically ventilated patients & nosocomial pneumonia, unless CI (*threatened cerebral perfusion pressure or intracranial hypertension*) ○ ↓ risk of aspiration • For Hyper/hypo delirium: Supportive & environmental measures, remove/reduce drug related causes, may consider antipsychotics (e.g., haloperidol, quetiapine).
U	Ulcer (stress) prophylaxis	• Initiate in mechanically ventilated patients • Also indicated for populations at ↑ risk of developing stress ulcers including mechanically ventilated > 48 hours, platelets < 50,000 or INR >1.5, on steroids, history of ulcers • Reassess whether prophylactic agent can be discontinued daily	• Add for the duration of hospital stay: Histamine receptor antagonists, proton pump inhibitors • Consider discontinuation of stress ulcer prophylaxis at time of discharge.
G	Glycemic control	• Select most appropriate insulin regimens or oral hypoglycemic drugs. • Identify drug-related causes such as glucocorticoids, propofol, atypical antipsychotics. • Achieve goal blood sugar of < 180 mg/dL.	• Consider dosing alterations: insulin: drip, basal-glargine, bolus-aspart

Notes: BP = blood pressure; MV = mechanical ventilation; LMWH = Low Molecular Weight Heparin; UFH = Unfractionated Heparin; CI = contraindication.
Based upon: Vincent JM. Give your patient a fast hug (at least) once a day. Crit Care Med 2005;33(6):1225–1229 & Mabasa VH, Malyuk DL, Weatherby EM, Chan A. A Standardized, Structured Approach to Identifying Drug-Related Problems in the Intensive Care Unit: FASTHUG-MAIDENS. CJHP 2011;64(5):366–369.

FASTHUG-MAIDENS: Approach to Identifying Drug-Related Problems (DRPs) & Aspects of Critical Care for Intensive Care Units (ICU) Pharmacists *(continued)*

SIDE 2—MAIDENS

Letter	Area of Care	Role	Examples
M	**Medication reconciliation**	• Review medications patient was receiving prior to admission. • Decide which drugs need to be restarted. • Assess medications upon admission, transfer, before discharge. • Identify discontinued medications for high risk of withdrawal symptoms (benzodiazepines, selective serotonin reuptake inhibitors).	• Ask patient "What medications are you currently using" & "How are you taking those medications?" & "Where are those medications filled?" • Ask patient about use of OTC products, such as aspirin, vitamins, pain relievers.
A	**Antibiotics/ Anti-infectives**	• Selecting optimal antimicrobial agent & de-escalating treatment. • Therapeutic drug monitoring	• If patient presents with sepsis or septic shock, start broad spectrum antibiotics. Once cultures/susceptibilities are available, modify therapy.
I	**Indication for meds**	• Review all regularly scheduled & as-needed medications daily. • Any medication that is no longer indicated should be discontinued.	• Identify indication for every medication on the medication list using PMH & HPI (e.g., antihypertensives for high BP)
D	**Drug Dosing**	• Suggest dose adjustments based on renal & hepatic function. • Therapeutic drug monitoring	• Monitor BUN, SCr, urine output for kidney function; AST, ALT, albumin, bilirubin for liver function; & adjust dose as needed.
E	**Electrolytes/ hematology/other laboratory results**	• Monitor patients for drug-related causes of abnormalities in electrolytes, hematology results, or laboratory values & discuss treatment alternatives.	• Refer to Fluid/Electrolytes Card in the Peripheral Brian.
N	**No drug interaction/ allergies/ duplications/ADRs**	• Identify clinically important potential & actual drug-drug, drug-food, drug-laboratory interactions.	• Common drugs to monitor for drug interactions/ADRs: Anticoagulants (e.g., warfarin), sedatives (e.g., midazolam), calcineurin inhibitors (e.g., tacrolimus, cyclosporine), macrolides (e.g., clarithromycin)
S	**Stop dates**	• Discuss appropriate duration of medications with other members of the health care team.	• Antimicrobial agents, glucocorticoids, opioid infusions

Notes: ADRs = adverse drug reactions; OTC = over-the-counter; PMH = past medical history; HPI = history of present illness; BP = blood pressure; BUN = blood urea nitrogen; SCr = serum creatinine; AST = aspartate aminotransferase; ALT = alanine aminotransferase.
Based upon: Mabasa VH, Malyuk DL, Weatherby EM, Chan A. A Standardized, Structured Approach to Identifying Drug-Related Problems in the Intensive Care Unit: FASTHUG-MAIDENS. CJHP 2011;64(5):366–369.

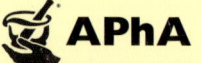
APhA

Pharmacy Mnemonics

INTERACTIONS

Warfarin Interactions: **ACADEMIC FACS**

Amiodarone; **C**iprofloxacin/levofloxacin; **A**spirin; **D**icloxacillin; **E**rythromycin (macrolides); **M**etronidazole (azole antifungals); **I**ndomethacin; **C**lofibrates; **F**ibrates; **A**llopurinol; **C**YP 2C9 inducers/inhibitors; **S**tatins

CYP-450 Enzyme Inhibitors: **BIG FACES.COM**

Bupropion; **I**traconazole/ketoconazole/fluconazole; **G**emfibrozil; **F**luoxetine/fluvoxamine; **A**miodarone; **C**iprofloxacin; **E**rythromycin/clarithromycin; **S**ulfamethoxazole-trimethorprim; **C**lopidogrel; **O**meprazole/esomeprazole; **M**etronidazole

CYP-450 Enzyme Inducers: **PS PORCS**

Phenytoin; **S**moking; **P**henobarbital; **O**xcarbazepine; **R**ifampin; **C**arbamazepine; **S**t. John's Wort

Simvastatin Increased Serum Levels: **ADIE**

Amiodarone; **D**iltiazem/verapamil; **I**traconazole; **E**rythromycin/clarithromycin

Prepared by Becky Petrik and Jeanine P. Abrons

SIDE EFFECTS

ACE Inhibitor: **CAPTOPRIL**

Cough; **A**ngioedema; **P**roteinuria/potassium excess; **T**aste changes; **O**rthostatic hypotension; **P**regnancy contraindication/pancreatitis; **R**enal failure/rash; **I**ndomethacin inhibition; **L**eukopenia/liver toxicity

Steroid: **BECLOMETHASONE**

Buffalo hump; **E**asy bruising; **C**ataracts; **L**arger appetite; **O**besity; **M**oonface; **E**motional changes (instability, euphoria); **T**hin arms and face; **H**yperglycemia/hypertension/hirsutism; **A**septic necrosis; **S**kin: striae, thinning, bruising (with topical preparations); **O**steoporosis; **N**egative nitrogen balance; **E**xtended wound healing

Morphine: **MORPHINES**

Miosis; **O**rthostatic hypotension; **R**espiratory depression; **P**neumonia; **H**istamine release/hormone changes; **I**nfrequency (constipation/urination); **N**ausea; **E**mesis; **S**edation

Increased Potassium (K^+) Levels: **K-BANK**

K^+ sparing diuretics/supplements; **B**eta blockers; **A**ngiotensin converting enzyme inhibitors (ACEI)/angiotensin receptor blockers (ARB); **N**onsteroidal anti-inflammatory drugs (NSAIDs); **K**idney disease

Prepared by Becky Petrik and Jeanine P. Abrons

Motivational Interviewing Techniques

Technique	Description	Example
Reframing/Rephrasing	• Strategy to help patients examine their perceptions in a different manner	• If a patient says people are always bothering me about quitting smoking – you could reframe to: Those people seem to care about you a lot.
Open-ended Questions	• Questions that a patient cannot answer yes or no to, but require an explanation	• Questions that begin with who; what; when; where; how • What questions do you have?
Reflective Listening → Paraphrasing	• Listening carefully to your patients; really hearing what they are saying & allowing the patient to be the focus • Varying levels of depth may be used	• Statements can be used: You are not quite sure that you are ready to make a change, but you are aware that your current behavior may negatively impact your health or it's been tough
Restating	• Simply restate what the patient has said	• Patient says "I'm frustrated." You say: "I understand, you are frustrated."
Readiness Ruler	• Scale from 1 to 7 • Asking patient how important the change is to him or her • First establish that it is of some importance (See example) • Next, establish that there is room for improvement (See example)	• Why a 3 & not a 1? • What would it take to move you from a 3 to a 7?
Modified Envelope Technique	• Helps the patient to identify their primary reason or focus for change	• If there was one thing that would motivate you to change, what would it be?

Prepared by Jeanine P. Abrons

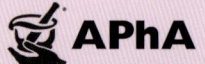

Pharmacists' Patient Care Process

Pharmacists' Patient Care Process

Pharmacists use a patient-centered approach in collaboration with other providers on the health care team to optimize patient health and medication outcomes.

Using principles of evidence-based practice, pharmacists:

Collect
The pharmacist assures the collection of the necessary subjective and objective information about the patient in order to understand the relevant medical/medication history and clinical status of the patient.

Assess
The pharmacist assesses the information collected and analyzes the clinical effects of the patient's therapy in the context of the patient's overall health goals in order to indentify and prioritize problems and achieve optimal care.

Plan
The pharmacist develops an individualized patient-centered care plan, in collaboration with other health care professionals and the patient or caregiver that is evidence based and cost effective.

Implement
The pharmacist implements the care plan in collaboration with other health care professionals and the patient or caregiver.

Follow-up: Monitor and Evaluate
The pharmacist monitors and evaluates the effectiveness of the care plan and modifies the plan in collaboration with other health care professionals and the patient or caregiver as needed.

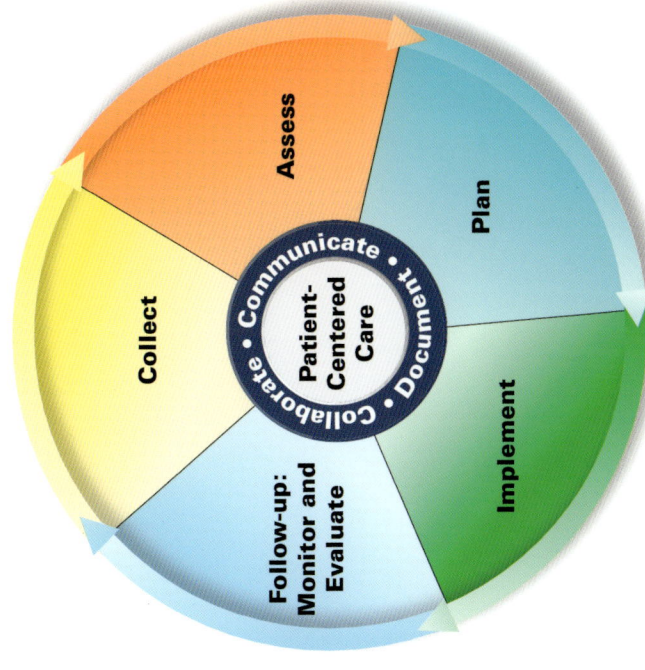

Source: Joint Commission of Pharmacy Practitioners, 2014